# The Fatigue
## • and •
# Fibromyalgia
# Solution

AVERY

*a member of Penguin Group (USA) Inc.*

*New York*

AVERY

Published by the Penguin Group
Penguin Group (USA) Inc., 375 Hudson Street,
New York, New York 10014, USA

USA · Canada · UK · Ireland · Australia
New Zealand · India · South Africa · China

Penguin Books Ltd, Registered Offices: 80 Strand, London WC2R 0RL, England
For more information about the Penguin Group visit penguin.com

Most Avery books are available at special quantity discounts for bulk purchase
for sales promotions, premiums, fund-raising, and educational needs. Special books
or book excerpts also can be created to fit specific needs. For details, write
Penguin Group (USA) Inc. Special Markets, 375 Hudson Street, New York, NY 10014.

ISBN 978-1-58333-514-7

Printed in the United States of America
3   5   7   9   10   8   6   4   2

*Book design by Meighan Cavanaugh*

Neither the publisher nor the author is engaged in rendering professional advice or services to the individual
reader. The ideas, procedures, and suggestions contained in this book are not intended as a substitute
for consulting with your physician. All matters regarding your health require medical supervision.
Neither the author nor the publisher shall be liable or responsible for any loss or damage
allegedly arising from any information or suggestion in this book.

While the author has made every effort to provide accurate telephone numbers, Internet addresses, and other
contact information at the time of publication, neither the publisher nor the author assumes any responsibility
for errors, or for changes that occur after publication. Further, the publisher does not have any control over
and does not assume any responsibility for author or third-party websites or their content.

# The Fatigue
· and ·
# Fibromyalgia
# Solution

THE ESSENTIAL GUIDE TO OVERCOMING

CHRONIC FATIGUE AND FIBROMYALGIA,

· · · **MADE EASY!** · · ·

Jacob Teitelbaum, M.D.

*To Laurie, my beautiful lady, my best friend, my wife,*
*and the love of my life, who always continues to inspire me;*
*my children, David, Amy, Shannon, Brittany, and Kelly,*
*who already seem to know so much of what I'm trying to learn;*
*my beautiful grandchildren, Payton, Bryce, and Emma;*
*my mother, Sabina, and father, David,*
*whose unconditional love made this book possible;*
*the memories of Drs. Janet Travell, Hugh Riordan, and*
*Billie Crook, who were the pioneers in this field;*
*and to my patients, who have taught me more*
*than I can ever hope to teach them.*

# *Acknowledgments*

So many special people helped make this book possible that I cannot possibly list them all. In truth, I have created nothing new; I have simply synthesized the wonderful work done by an army of hardworking and courageous physicians and healers.

I would like to extend my sincerest thanks to, first and foremost, my wife, Laurie, whose insights continue to inspire new ideas in my understanding of chronic fatigue syndrome, fibromyalgia, and healing in general. In addition to being incredibly patient with me while I wrote this book, and planting the seeds for many of the concepts I discuss, she was the first to convince me (translation: pound into my thick manly skull) that I needed to heed my readers and keep this book short and simple. So my special thanks and love to you, Laurie, who, like wives everywhere, often triggers the insights that help their men to grow!

Thank you also to:

My staff. Their hard work, compassion, and dedication (and, I must admit, patience with me) are what made my work possible. I want to especially thank my office manager and patient educator, Cheryl Alberto, who is infinitely patient with me no matter how much chaos I create, and makes sure that everything happens correctly, while I am off doing the easy things like writing books; Denise Haire and Stacey Soltis, who keep things flowing smoothly for our patients; and Sherry Gracie, who makes sure that people get their supplements quickly and accurately.

The Anne Arundel Medical Center librarian, Joyce Miller. Over the last thirty-two years, I have often wondered when she would politely tell me to stop asking for so many studies. So far, she has not. In fact, she always smiles when I ask her for more. Truly an angel!

Bren Jacobson, Dr. Alan Weiss, and Jain Vaughn, who keep me intellectually, emotionally, and spiritually honest while reminding me to keep my sense of humor.

My wonderful and dedicated publicists, Dean Draznin, Diane Chojnowski, Terri Slater, and the rest of the Dean Draznin gang; and to Richard Crouse, my Webmaster, who simply and easily makes everything I ask for happen—over and over again!

These are but a few of my teammates in making effective treatment and health available to everyone. For those I didn't mention, I thank you all!

The publishers at Avery/Penguin, and my superb editor, Marisa Vigilante, who worked closely with me to make this book excellent. Also to Rudy Shur, my first publisher and a man with an ongoing vision.

My many teachers, the real heroes and heroines in their fields, whose names could fill this book. Especially William Crook, Max Boverman, Brugh Joy, Janet Travell, Hugh Riordan, William Jefferies, Hal Blatman, Robert Ivker, and Alan Gaby.

The many chronic fatigue syndrome and fibromyalgia support groups. These are easily the best patient support groups I have ever seen.

And finally, God and the universe, for the guidance and infinite blessings I have been given and for using me as an instrument for healing.

# Contents

# Introduction

Ready to feel great? It's not that hard to do!

If you're like most people, you wish you had more energy. How often do you meet somebody who has all the energy they'd like, with even some left over to spare?

I'm one of those people. But it wasn't always this way. I came down with chronic fatigue syndrome and fibromyalgia (CFS/FMS) back in 1975, before these syndromes even had a name. I had to drop out of medical school, and was homeless and sleeping in parks for much of the next year. While I was homeless, a remarkable thing happened. I met numerous health practitioners from a wide variety of disciplines, and I learned what I needed to do to be able to recover and return to medical school. I met so many health practitioners that it was as if the universe put a "Homeless Medical School" sign on my park bench! This experience also inspired me to continue exploring how to optimize energy production and vitality over the last thirty-seven years.

So whether you have day-to-day fatigue and are simply looking to feel great, or have chronic fatigue syndrome or fibromyalgia (CFS/

FMS) and need "intensive care" for your energy crisis, this book is for you. It will teach you, in a simple and easy way, how to dramatically optimize your energy using the SHINE protocol, which stands for Sleep, Hormones, Infections, Nutrition, and Exercise as able.

For most of you with day-to-day fatigue, a few simple tips in each of these areas will be enough to leave you feeling like a powerhouse. We will start off each chapter with these basics. We will then finish off each area by discussing SHINE Intensive Care, describing more advanced and powerful treatments for those with very severe fatigue or CFS and fibromyalgia. These treatments have been shown in our published research to increase energy an outstanding average of 91 percent.

As research into CFS/FMS (the term I will use throughout the book for chronic fatigue syndrome and fibromyalgia syndrome) rapidly expanded, so did the size of each edition of my earlier book, *From Fatigued to Fantastic!* The previous edition was almost four times the length of the first one, which I wrote eighteen years ago! Many really appreciated the depth of information. Many others, especially given the severity of their brain fog, found it overwhelming and asked if I could write a really simple and easy version of the book. And my wife, Laurie, has been encouraging me to do this for almost a decade.

So here it is . . .

*The Fatigue and Fibromyalgia Solution*—MADE EASY!

For those who are looking to understand these illnesses easily, and simply learn how to get your lives back, this book is for you. It quickly will allow you to learn what you need to know to get well. After reading and applying what you learn in this book, you may find that you are then ready to take the next step. If so, I invite you to read *From*

*Fatigued to Fantastic!* for even more in-depth and comprehensive information, along with hundreds of references for the studies this information is based on. The citations for studies that came out after *From Fatigued to Fantastic!* can be found at www.vitality101.com.

This book is also excellent for readers without CFS/FMS who simply want more energy and vitality, or need help with sleep, hormonal problems, candida, and nutritional support. Meanwhile, for those who have read the earlier textbook-length versions and simply want to get up to date on the newest information without wading through 150,000 words, this book is also for you.

So would you like 91 percent more energy without having to read a 450-page textbook with small print?

Here's how.

# PART 1

# Your Body's Energy Crisis

# 1.

# Why We Have a Modern-Day Energy Crisis

Some of you may remember a disaster film released in 2000 called *The Perfect Storm*, in which circumstances conspired to create a massive, ship-sinking storm. Unfortunately, there is now a "perfect storm" for the creation of an exhaustion epidemic, with seven major factors coming together to overwhelm people.

These energy drains include:

1. *Widespread nutritional deficiencies.* With 18 percent of our diet's calories coming from sugar, another 18 percent from white flour, and loads of saturated fat, almost half of the modern diet has had the vitamins, minerals, and other key nutrients (except for calories) processed away. This is why we are facing high-calorie malnutrition, with people who are both obese and malnourished, for the first time in human history. Dozens of nutrients are critical for our energy-producing machinery, and without these, fats and other calories cannot be converted into energy. This leaves people both overweight and exhausted.

2. *Sleep deficiency.* Until 130 years ago, when Thomas Edison invented the lightbulb, the average night's sleep was nine hours a night. Now, with television, computers, and both the stresses and conveniences of modern life, we are down to an average of only six and three-quarters hours of sleep a night. This is like a 30 percent pay cut to your body.

3. *An overwhelmed immune system.* Where there used to be none for most of human history, we now have over 85,000 new chemicals added to our environment. These are all new to our immune system, which has to figure out how to handle each and every one of them. This by itself can leave our immune systems on overdrive. In addition, modern life also suffers from an ill-fated combination of poor digestion of proteins caused by the destruction of food enzymes during food processing, combined with "leaky gut" from candida and other bowel infections. This mix results in food proteins being absorbed into the blood before they are completely digested. These then have to be treated like foreign invaders, triggering food allergies and immune exhaustion, as well as a marked increase in autoimmune diseases such as lupus.

4. In addition to the other stresses faced by the immune system, the introduction of antibiotics and acid blockers has dramatically changed the mix of bacteria in our gut. There are more bacteria in the colon than cells in the whole rest of our body, so overgrowth with toxic bacteria is a big problem and can result in a massive energy drain. This is why probiotics, which add good bacteria back to your system, are becoming so popular.

5. *Hormonal deficiencies.* The most common cause of low thyroid (Hashimoto's thyroiditis) and adrenal destruction (Addison's disease) is autoimmune disease, where the body mistakes the gland for an outside invader and attacks it. In addition, increased stress suppresses a major hormonal control center called the hypothalamus (a key "circuit breaker" we will talk about in the next chapter), which controls hormone function. High stress can also exhaust our stress-handling adrenal glands. The thyroid and adrenal glands are critical not only for the production of energy but also for our ability to handle stress.

6. *Decreased exercise and sunshine.* Sometimes, it seems that all the exercise that some people get these days is pushing down on the gas pedal and their television remote control buttons. This causes deconditioning. Meanwhile, the lack of sunshine from not being outside exercising, as well as the misguided medical advice to avoid sunshine, is causing an epidemic of vitamin D deficiency. Vitamin D is critical for regulating immune function, and deficiency is one more stress that results in decreased energy by triggering autoimmune illness while increasing the risk of cancer and infections.

7. *Increased life stresses.* The speed of modern life is increasing dramatically. It used to be that if you wanted to send somebody a letter, it was delivered by pony express and could take weeks to get a response. Now with e-mails, it takes minutes. In addition, I remember the good old days when the mantra of Madison Avenue advertising executives was "Sex sells." Now it's "Fear sells." Where TV and news stations used to focus on romance and comedy, now

they seem to focus instead on trying to scare people to death, and rather than giving today's news, they invent "today's crisis."

The good news? As each generation faces new health challenges, we also develop the tools needed to handle them. Our generation is no exception. Modern medicine has created many wonderful inventions. The bad news? Unfortunately, we also face a problem these days, with medical economics often winning out over medical sanity. Fortunately, knowledge is power, and the information in this book will teach you what you need to know to get well NOW!

## A MODERN HEALTH-CARE CHALLENGE

A curious thing happened during the rigorous process I went through to become a physician. By the time I completed my formal training, I presumed that if an important treatment existed for an illness, I had been taught about it in medical school. I understood, of course, that physicians needed to continue their education to stay abreast of new information and treatments. But I felt sure that if someone claimed he or she could effectively treat a "nontreatable" disease, that person was a quack.

I was wrong.

Having spent over thirty-five years and countless hours exploring the scientific literature, I've been shocked to find that research shows that natural remedies frequently work better than prescriptions. Meanwhile, the natural remedies come with fewer side effects and a much lower price tag. I've also learned that often natural remedies and prescription drugs work better together than either one alone. Overall, I find people do best starting with natural therapies, saving the medications for cases where they are needed. It also shocked me to realize that most physicians' continuing medical education is paid for almost entirely by the pharmaceutical industry and medical equipment suppliers—and can be accurately described as "slick marketing masquerading as scientific educational activities." This means that the only things that most physicians learn about after medical school are what is most profitable to pharmaceutical companies—which certainly does not include most natural therapies.

Dr. Marcia Angell, past editor of the prestigious *New England Journal of Medicine*, described what is happening in modern medicine very succinctly (and frighteningly) when she said:

"It is simply no longer possible to believe much of the clinical research that is published, or to rely on the judgment of trusted physicians or authoritative medical guidelines. I take no pleasure in this conclusion, which I reached slowly and reluctantly over my two decades as an editor of *The New England Journal of Medicine*."

Working as a patient advocate, my preference is to offer you whatever the science and clinical experience shows is most effective, safest, and most economical. To maintain objectivity, I long ago decided to take no money from any natural or pharmaceutical product companies, and 100 percent of the royalties for products I design are donated to charity. This allows me to recommend and carry what I find to be the best products from many companies, and to give unabashedly both natural and prescription options either a thumbs-up or a "raspberry," as they deserve. It also makes it easier to offer people the best of natural and standard medicine—which the late Dr. Hugh Riordan called "comprehensive medicine." Basically, this means having the entire health "tool kit" available instead of only a hammer.

For most people with day-to-day fatigue, simple natural therapies can be dramatically effective at optimizing energy. We will start each treatment chapter with foundation therapies to optimize energy production for everyone, even those with mild to moderate fatigue.

But some people do have more severe problems, sometimes requiring medications. This is the situation that occurs in people who have a very severe energy crisis, where they essentially "blow a fuse" and develop chronic fatigue syndrome and fibromyalgia (abbreviated CFS/FMS throughout the book). In these cases, additional energy "intensive care" is needed, and it is discussed at the end of each treatment chapter.

The approach you will learn about in *The Fatigue and Fibromyalgia Solution* is well grounded in the scientific literature and clinical experience, and the references for hundreds of medical studies supporting what I discuss are readily available in earlier books and articles I've written (we've left these references out as part of keeping it simple). Instead of just throwing a medication at each symptom you have, the approach we discuss in this book will treat the problems' underlying, perpetuating factors and root causes, so you can heal.

So let's take a look at what chronic fatigue syndrome and fibromyalgia (CFS/FMS) are and what they feel like. Although there are literally dozens of symptoms present in CFS/FMS, many of these can also be present in other conditions. A simple way to distinguish CFS/FMS from other causes of exhaustion? If you don't also have insomnia, you likely don't have CFS/FMS and can feel free to skip the next chapter. Those of you who have the paradox of having severe insomnia despite being exhausted likely have CFS/FMS, even if you have other conditions such as lupus or rheumatoid arthritis, and this next chapter is for you.

# 2.

# What Are Chronic Fatigue Syndrome and Fibromyalgia?

Exhausted, widespread pain, brain fog, and can't sleep? If you answered yes, you're one of over 12 million Americans, and one of over 100 million people worldwide, with a chronic fatigue syndrome or fibromyalgia–related process. Over the past few decades, the incidence of chronic fatigue syndrome (CFS) and fibromyalgia (FMS) has exploded and is now present in approximately 12 to 24 million Americans! Meanwhile, one out of every four Americans suffers with inadequately treated chronic pain and 31 percent of adults are *chronically* fatigued.

People with CFS/FMS are like the tip of an iceberg that is rapidly coming to surface. As the numbers grow, these conditions will become increasingly hard to ignore.

So you are not alone. Even if sometimes you feel that way.

Put simply, chronic fatigue syndrome and fibromyalgia (CFS/FMS) represent a severe energy crisis in your body, where you essentially blow a fuse. Just like there are many ways to blow a circuit breaker in your home, there are many ways to do so in your body, causing CFS and FMS. In this book, we will teach you how to get rid of these energy leaks while turbocharging energy production. This way, the circuit breaker kicks back on, and your body will feel like it is coming back to life.

Let's start with the basics.

# Making the Diagnosis—the Standard Way

There are differing definitions that are used clinically and in research. Just to offer an idea of these, I have included three common ones. They are pretty irrelevant for your day-to-day care, so feel free to skip them:

1. The 1994 U.S. CDC (Centers for Disease Control) definition for CFS—a definition with which I am wholly *un*impressed.

## CDC CRITERIA FOR CHRONIC FATIGUE SYNDROME

A case of chronic fatigue syndrome is defined by the presence of the following:

1. Clinically evaluated, unexplained, persistent, or relapsing chronic fatigue that is of new or definite onset (has not been lifelong); is not the result of ongoing exertion; is not substantially alleviated by rest; and results in substantial reduction in previous levels of occupational, educational, social, or personal activities.
2. Concurrent occurrence of four or more of the following symptoms, all of which must have persisted or recurred

*(continued)*

during six or more consecutive months of illness and must not have predated the fatigue:

A. Self-reported impairment in short-term memory or concentration severe enough to cause substantial reduction in previous levels of occupational, educational, social, or personal activities

B. Sore throat

C. Tender cervical [neck] or axillary [underarm] lymph nodes

D. Muscle pain

E. Multijoint pain without joint swelling or redness

F. Headaches of a new type, pattern, or severity

G. Unrefreshing sleep

H. Postexertional malaise lasting more than twenty-four hours

Adapted from *Annals of Internal Medicine* 121 (14 December 1994). Used with permission.

2. The old 1990 ACR (American College of Rheumatology) diagnostic criteria for fibromyalgia. This required a person to have persistent widespread pain, and eleven of eighteen tender points on the tender point exam, which most doctors have absolutely no clue how to do.

3. 2011 ACR modified diagnostic criteria for fibromyalgia, which no longer uses the tender point exam and is a marked improvement. The 2010 ACR criteria are in more common use, but I consider them unnecessarily vague and recommend the 2011 criteria below.

## 2011 Modified ACR Fibromyalgia Diagnostic Criteria

A patient satisfies diagnostic criteria for fibromyalgia if the following conditions are met:

1. Widespread pain index (WPI) ≥7 and symptom severity (SS) scale score ≥5 or WPI 3 to 6 and SS scale score ≥9.
2. Symptoms have been present at a similar level for at least three months.
3. The patient does not have a disorder that would otherwise explain the pain.

Take this test and add:

1. _____ WPI: Circle each area where you've had pain over the last week. Count these (score will be between 0 and 19).

| Shoulder girdle, left | Hip (buttock, trochanter), left | Jaw, left | Upper back |
|---|---|---|---|
| Shoulder girdle, right | Hip (buttock, trochanter), right | Jaw, right | Lower back |
| Upper arm, left | Upper leg, left | Chest | Neck |
| Upper arm, right | Upper leg, right | Abdomen | |
| Lower arm, left | Lower leg, left | | |
| Lower arm, right | Lower leg, right | | |

2. SS scale score: For each of the three symptoms below, score its
severity over the past week, using the following scale:

| 0 = | No problem |
|-----|------------|
| 1 = | Slight or mild problems, generally mild or intermittent |
| 2 = | Moderate, considerable problems, often present and/or at a moderate level |
| 3 = | Severe, pervasive, continuous, life-disturbing problems |

_____ Fatigue (score 0 to 3)
_____ Waking unrefreshed (score 0 to 3)
_____ Cognitive symptoms ("brain fog") (score 0 to 3)

Then add <u>JUST 1 point</u> for each of the following three symptoms
that have occurred during the previous six months:

_____ headaches (score 0 to 1)
_____ pain or cramps in lower abdomen (score 0 to 1)
_____ depression (score 0 to 1)

_____ Total SS scale score (adding the six items above). The final score
is between 0 and 12.

---

Technically, the 2011 ACR modified diagnostic criteria are not
supposed to be used by the patient, but only by doctors. I don't believe that this limitation is really necessary. Happily, though, in real
life there is a much simpler way to tell if you have a CFS/FMS-related
process and are likely to improve with SHINE treatments.

# Telling If You Have CFS and/or Fibromyalgia—Made Easy

Simply answer these four questions:

1. Do you have severe fatigue, along with insomnia and perhaps brain fog?
2. Have you been checked by your doctor, and no other overt cause was found (being told you're depressed or crazy because the doctor was clueless doesn't count)?
3. Has it lasted over three months?
   If yes to these three, you likely have CFS until proven otherwise.
4. Do you also have widespread pain?

If yes, then you also have fibromyalgia.
In most cases, it is that simple.

Another name for a condition with related symptoms is myalgic encephalomyelitis. This diagnosis tends to be used more in Canada and Europe. Although there are differences in how they are defined, and every case is different, I consider CFS, fibromyalgia, and myalgic encephalomyelitis (ME) to be related and overlapping conditions that all respond well to the treatments discussed in this book, so I use the term CFS/FMS to refer to all of these.

**A QUICK TIP**

Though in most cases CFS and fibromyalgia are two names for the same condition, because of current politics and the social stigma attached to the diagnosis of CFS, you will generally do better to use the fibromyalgia label instead of chronic fatigue syndrome. Some good news from an unexpected quarter? The pharmaceutical industry is spending nearly $270 million a year on advertising to make the diagnosis of fibromyalgia medically and socially acceptable, so it can create a larger market for its three new FDA-approved fibromyalgia medications.

# What Chronic Fatigue Syndrome and Fibromyalgia Feel Like

Chronic fatigue syndrome and fibromyalgia occur in varying degrees of severity, ranging from moderately disruptive to leaving some people bedridden. And no, these are *not* happening because you are depressed or "you're getting older." They're happening because you have CFS/FMS!

There are dozens of symptoms that can be seen with CFS/FMS. Doctors not familiar with the illness, even excellent physicians, have difficulty making sense of this wide array of symptoms, so their reactions may have left you and your family confused and concerned. Some especially clueless physicians may have even implied that since *they* don't know what's wrong, *you* must be crazy!

So let's clear this up for you right now!

The most common complaints among chronic fatigue and fibro-myalgia patients include:

• *Overwhelming fatigue.* Most people with CFS/FMS are fatigued most of the time. Occasionally, they experience short periods during which they feel better. However, after several hours or days of feeling energetic, they typically crash back down into severe fatigue.

Often, CFS patients wake up feeling tired and spend the day that way. Oddly, they often have the most energy between 10 p.m. and 4 a.m., in part because their day/night cycles are reversed. In addition, too much exercise often makes the fatigue worse. When CFS/FMS patients try to exercise, they feel worse that day and as if they were "hit by a truck" the next. If you have CFS/FMS, this "postexertional fatigue" occurs because you can't make enough energy to condition during exercise, simply depleting your energy instead. This causes further deconditioning and discouragement. A better approach is to walk as much as you can, but only to the point where you feel "good tired" after the exercise and better the next day. After approximately ten weeks of gentle, slow walking to begin reconditioning, while doing the treatments discussed in this book, most people find that they can start to increase their walking by up to one minute a day as their energy levels increase. Once you can walk for about an hour a day, then you can start slowly increasing the intensity of exercise. See chapter 8, "E—Exercise, as Able."

• *Severe insomnia.* People with CFS/FMS are lucky to be able to sleep five hours a night despite being exhausted. Meanwhile, it's like an alarm clock goes off every night between two and four in the morning, waking up everybody with these conditions. Restless leg syndrome and sleep apnea are also much more common in people with CFS/FMS.

- *Brain fog.* People with CFS/FMS often suffer from poor short-term memory and difficulty with word finding and word substitution. Sometimes you may even have to think for a moment to remember your children's names! About one-third of people will also have rare, brief episodes of disorientation, lasting thirty seconds to two minutes. These most often happen when taking an exit ramp while driving or making a turn in a store aisle. It can feel frightening, but it is not dangerous and passes quickly.

Brain fog is one of the most frustrating symptoms for some people and is often the scariest. Many people are afraid that they are developing Alzheimer's disease. But this is not the case. A simple way to differentiate between brain fog and dementia is that with brain fog, you may constantly forget where you left the keys. With Alzheimer's, however, you may forget how to *use* your keys. They are not the same, and the brain fog also routinely improves, and often resolves, by using the SHINE protocol.

- *Achiness and pain.* Achiness in both muscles and joints is also common, and may progress to nerve pain as well. Initially, it feels like you have achy muscles in many different parts of your body. As you shift positions and how you carry your weight in response to the pain, the pain may move around to different areas over time. In the beginning, this pain is predominantly from tight muscles and is associated with tender knots in the muscles called trigger points (where the belly of the shortened muscle bunches up). These feel like tender marbles when someone gives you a massage.

As the condition progresses, some people develop numbness or tingling in their hands or feet (paresthesias and carpal tunnel syndrome), and sometimes burning/shooting pains (nerve pain or neuropathy). Sometimes the skin is even sensitive to touch (called allodynia). All of these pains can be effectively treated and are discussed in chapter 9, "Natural and Prescription Pain Relief."

• **Increased thirst.** Because of hormonal problems, people with chronic fatigue and fibromyalgia often have decreased ability to hold on to salt and water, which increases urine output and thirst. A classic description of CFS/FMS is that you "drink like a fish and pee like a racehorse." Drinking a lot of water and *increasing* salt intake becomes important and will help you feel better. As we discuss regarding low adrenal function in chapter 5, "H—Hormonal Support: Optimizing Adrenal, Thyroid, Testosterone, and Estrogen Function," trying to restrict salt when you have CFS/FMS is a quick way to "crash and burn." When people ask me how many glasses of water to drink a day, I tell them a much better approach is simply to check your mouth and lips. If they are dry, you are thirsty and need to drink more water.

It is important to note that dry eyes and dry mouth that do not improve when you drink more water (called sicca syndrome) are also common. These symptoms can often be resolved by taking fish-oil

(Vectomega) and sea buckthorn oil (Hydra 7) supplements, B vitamins, and magnesium.

- *Frequent infections.* Many CFS/FMS patients have:

  1. Recurrent respiratory infections, sore throats, and swollen glands and seem to catch every cold that's going around. This tends to resolve with adrenal support (see chapter 5).
  2. Chronic sinusitis, nasal congestion. and postnasal drip. This is most often caused by candida/yeast.
  3. Digestive disorders, including gas, cramps, and alternating diarrhea and constipation. These are usually attributed to spastic colon (irritable bowel syndrome). Spastic colon means that you have these symptoms and your doctor does not know why. In CFS/FMS, these are usually triggered by bowel infections, especially candida, and improve with treatment.
  4. Continuing body-wide flu-like symptoms. These patients often have reactivation of an old virus.

- *Allergies and sensitivities.* CFS/FMS patients often have a history of being sensitive to many foods and medications. I find that food sensitivities and other sensitivities usually improve when the adrenal insufficiency and yeast or parasitic overgrowth are treated. Desensitization techniques such as NAET (Nambudripad's Allergy Elimination Technique) can also be very helpful in more severe cases (more about this in chapter 6).

- *Anxiety and depression.* Approximately 12 percent of people with CFS have marked anxiety, sometimes with palpitations, sweating, and other signs of panic. Metabolically, CFS/FMS sometimes leaves people more prone to hyperventilation as well as a rapid resting pulse. These symptoms, too, often improve with treatment. In addition, CFS/FMS does not make you immune to depression. Unfortunately, some physicians will simply label a person as depressed if they can't figure out what is wrong with them, instead of honestly saying they don't know. It is abusive for a doctor to tell a patient, "I don't know what is wrong with you, so you're crazy!" If your doctor says this, he or she is unlikely to be able to help you and you need to find another physician (see chapter 13). Fortunately, this kind of nonsense is becoming less common as physicians are learning more about these illnesses.

So how can you tell if you are depressed? Well, for starters, ask yourself! Research shows that simply asking is as reliable as fancy depression scales. Another way to tell? Do you have many interests? If you have a lot of interests but are frustrated that you don't have the energy to do them, you are probably not clinically depressed.

- *Weight gain.* Studies done in our research center show that people with CFS and fibromyalgia gain an average of thirty-two pounds with their illness. I suspect this occurs because of changes in metabolism caused by low thyroid function, yeast overgrowth, a deficiency of acetyl-L-carnitine, insulin resistance, immune dysfunction, and poor sleep. Many patients are thrilled not only to feel better and have their pain go away with treatment but also to find their weight dropping (see chapter 12).

- *Decreased libido.* When asked how their libido is, most people with CFS/FMS (73 percent in one of our studies) answer, "What libido?" In addition to pain and a general "yucky" feeling, hormonal deficiencies also contribute to this symptom. However, libido often improves with treatment, though it may take six to nine months.

• Many other common symptoms include: occasional shortness of breath (not with exercise), non-exertional chest pain (usually benign chest wall muscle tenderness, but check with your doctor to be safe), occasional dizziness on standing, and even bladder and pelvic pain. We'll discuss these more later on in the book.

You may have recognized yourself as you read through this list. If you did, please be assured that you are not alone. You are part of a large group of over 100 million people worldwide.

## What Causes CFS and Fibromyalgia?

Poor sleep, poor nutrition, an overwhelmed immune system, hormone system malfunctioning, and the increased speed of modern life are all contributing to people "blowing a fuse." But why are there so many diverse symptoms?

### THE ROLE OF THE HYPOTHALAMIC CIRCUIT BREAKER

As we noted above, the energy crisis in CFS/FMS causes people to have a major control center, called the hypothalamus, go into hibernation mode. I call this "blowing a fuse." I grew up with a fuse box in our home, and when I came down with CFS, it felt exactly like I blew a fuse. So this is the expression that I will use here. But I recognize that fuse boxes have largely disappeared. Nowadays, instead, what occurs is tripping a circuit breaker. So I will use the expressions "blowing a fuse" and "tripping a circuit breaker" interchangeably.

The hypothalamus, a critical control center in the brain, goes off-line first during an energy crisis because it uses more energy for its size than any other area in your body. This is because it controls so many different functions, as I'll discuss below.

Fortunately, no damage is done to the hypothalamus during this process. When energy production is restored, so is hypothalamic function.

## THE HYPOTHALAMUS—A MAJOR CONTROL CENTER

Understanding the four key functions controlled by the hypothalamus explains most of the symptoms seen in CFS/FMS. These functions are:

1. *Sleep.* The hypothalamus is a major sleep control center. When it goes off-line, people get horrible insomnia despite being exhausted. This is why the inability to sleep despite being exhausted is such a good marker distinguishing CFS/FMS from fatigue with other causes.

2. *Hormonal function.* The hypothalamus controls our body's entire hormonal system through the pituitary gland, which is located right below the hypothalamus. Because of this,

*(continued)*

people with CFS/FMS have symptoms of low thyroid (tired, achy, brain fog, and weight gain), low adrenal (irritability when hungry and crashing during stress), and low estrogen or testosterone.

3. *Autonomic nervous system regulation.* This is what controls blood pressure, pulse, sweating, and bowel function. This is why we often see low blood pressure, rapid pulse, unusual sweating patterns, and acid reflux.

4. *Temperature regulation.* Although you may sometimes feel feverish, you'll find that your temperature is usually below 98.6°F. In fact, in people with CFS and fibromyalgia, a temperature over 99 usually reflects a fever.

## SO HOW CAN I TELL WHAT "BLEW MY FUSE"?

Often, the problem that caused the initial stress is long gone (e.g., an auto accident), and the treatments in this book will simply turn the circuit breaker back on. In other cases, it will be important to avoid what caused you to blow your fuse in the first place. For example, if you get well so you can go back to a toxic job that made you sick in the first place, you will likely simply blow a fuse again. (We'll talk about how to avoid this in chapter 11, "Am I Crazy?: Understanding the Mind-Body Connection.")

Below are some of the most common triggers to consider.

### IF YOUR ILLNESS BEGAN SUDDENLY:

1. Viral, parasitic, or antibiotic-sensitive infections
2. Injury (even mild "fender bender" accidents)

3. Pregnancy (usually beginning soon after the baby is born)
4. Toxic exposures (especially if others around you also got sick)

**IF YOUR ILLNESS CAME ON GRADUALLY, CONSIDER:**

1. Yeast (candida) overgrowth—especially if you have sinusitis or nasal congestion and/or spastic colon
2. Hormonal deficiencies (even if your blood tests are normal)— especially low thyroid or low hormone levels due to peri-menopause
3. Chronic stress, including both at work and within relationships. These syndromes commonly affect hardworking "adrenaline junkies"
4. Autoimmune disorders (e.g., lupus, rheumatoid arthritis, Sjögren's syndrome)
5. Anything that disrupts sleep, including sleep apnea, restless leg syndrome, or a spouse who snores

If you think about blowing a fuse in your home, although it is annoying, it protects your home from burning down during a power surge. In the same way, I do not view CFS/FMS as the enemy. Rather, I see them as attempts on the body's part to protect itself from further harm and damage in the face of any of a number of overwhelming stresses.

I suspect that the root cause of the hypothalamic suppression can be found in the mitochondria, or the "energy furnaces" in the cells. The good news is that restoring adequate energy production using the SHINE treatments we'll discuss can jump-start your healing process by optimizing mitochondrial energy production and restoring function in your hypothalamic circuit breaker. There is no single magic bullet to get well, however. People who suffer from CFS/FMS usually have a combination of several different problems, and the exact combination varies considerably from individual to individual. It is important to look for and treat all of the factors simultaneously.

## SO WHY DO I HAVE PAIN?

When muscles do not have enough energy you might think that they would go loose and limp, but that is not the case. Think about writer's cramp, when your muscles stop getting enough energy. When this happens, the muscles become tight—often stiff as a board—and they will hurt. The multiple little painful knots (called trigger points) are the belly of the muscles where they have bunched up. As people feel pain from these knots, they start shifting their weight to take the strain off the uncomfortable areas. Unfortunately, this puts more strain on other areas, and the pain starts moving around your body.

In addition, when you're not able to get deep sleep, your muscles do not heal from the day's activities, and this also contributes to pain. Many of you have probably noticed that the few nights you can get a good night's sleep, the pain decreases.

To add insult to injury, once you develop chronic pain, the brain actually starts to amplify the pain, and the brain itself can then trigger the pain. This is called "central sensitization." Central sensitization is what you hear most about in discussions of fibromyalgia pain. This is not because it is the main problem. Instead, I suspect this is because the three FDA-approved medications for fibromyalgia target central sensitization. But this is just one modest piece of the pain process, with the key source and root cause of the pain being from the tight muscles.

In addition, chronic pain of many types can also commonly trigger a secondary nerve pain, called chronic inflammatory demyelinating polyneuropathy (CIDP), and low thyroid (despite normal lab tests) also increases the tendency of getting carpal tunnel syndrome (found in 45 percent of people with fibromyalgia). This is where tissue swelling compresses a nerve going through the wrist, causing numbness, tingling, and pain in your hands. This generally also goes away with thyroid and vitamin $B_6$ (see chapter 9, "Natural and Prescription Pain Relief").

Bottom line? You'll be amazed at how dramatically your pain can be decreased and usually eliminated as you get eight to nine hours of deep sleep a night, optimize thyroid function, restore energy production in your muscles (which is what this book is about), and stop sending excessive pain signals to your brain.

It never ceases to amaze me how quickly a case of fibromyalgia can resolve once the underlying problems are treated. In fact, the duration of the disease simply does not seem to affect how responsive it is to treatment. Two of the top authorities on muscle pain, the late and great Drs. Janet Travell and David Simons, devoted much of their life's work to studying muscle trigger points, and their research laid the foundation for much of what we discuss in this book.

## THE GOOD NEWS

The good news is that everything I have discussed above is treatable. The trick is to sort out which problems are most active in each individual and to treat them all. We certainly have much more to learn, but we already know enough to help most people reclaim their lives.

## IMPORTANT POINTS

- Chronic fatigue syndrome (CFS) is characterized by the paradox of inability to sleep despite being exhausted, brain fog, and, if fibromyalgia (FMS) is also present, widespread pain. You may have a variety of other symptoms as well. Common symptoms include increased thirst, weight gain, low libido, spastic colon, nasal congestion/sinusitis, and frequent infections.
- CFS and FMS occur when you expend more energy than you can make. This overloads your circuits, causing you to "blow a fuse" called the hypothalamus.
- Research shows that effective therapy is available for 91 percent of people with CFS/FMS by simply treating with the SHINE (Sleep, Hormones, Infections, Nutrition, and Exercise as able) protocol.

# 3.

# Create Your Individual
# Treatment Protocol

We've talked about why your body is having an energy crisis. Now let's talk about optimizing energy production and eliminating the things that are draining your body's fuel tank. We call this the SHINE protocol, which stands for the five main treatment areas:

1. Sleep
2. Hormonal deficiencies
3. Infections
4. Nutritional deficiencies
5. Exercise as able

In addition to powerfully helping regular fatigue, our published, placebo-controlled study (see Appendix B) shows that when you treat these five building blocks of health, 91 percent of people with CFS/FMS, the worst type of energy crisis, improved their energy levels and decreased their pain—with an average 75 percent improvement in quality of life at three months and 90 percent at two years. This reflects what I see in day-to-day practice, treating people from all over the world.

So there is good reason to be hopeful.

Part 2 will go into the specifics of each of the five SHINE treatment areas, and in Part 3 you'll learn how to overcome other problems, such as chronic pain, weight gain, and mind-body issues. Several appendices at the end of the book offer additional or supporting information, including a treatment checklist that you can fill in as you read the book, to help you tailor an energy-optimizing protocol to your specific case.

Your doctor may not be familiar with the research on effective treatment of chronic fatigue and fibromyalgia. If this is the case, you may want to show your doctor the abstracts of two of my clinical studies that are available in Appendix B. The full text of several of the studies done by our research center using the treatments discussed in this book can also be found at www.vitality101.com. Feel free to download the studies from the Web site and give your physicians a copy.

If you are looking for a new doctor, turn to chapter 13 for more information on what to look for and how to choose a practitioner. In addition, I also personally treat patients worldwide, doing consultations by phone or in person. See www.endfatigue.com for a worldwide Practitioner Referral List or for information on making an appointment with me.

If you finish the book and find yourself wishing for more information:

A. Check my Web sites.
At www.endfatigue.com:

1. Sign up for my free e-mail newsletter so you can stay on the cutting edge of new research information.
2. Do the free online "Energy Analysis Program" that can analyze your symptoms and, if available, even your pertinent lab tests, to help you tailor an energy optimization regimen specific to your case.

At www.vitality101.com:

1. See hundreds of articles on CFS, FMS, and other health conditions.

B. Read my book *From Fatigued to Fantastic!* It is much more complex and detailed and offers a wealth of information, being more like a textbook. It has been the number one most read book on CFS and FMS—ever! But people kept asking me to make this simple version . . .

## How to Follow the SHINE Protocol

As you read this book, you'll find questions at the end of many chapters; answer the questions and check off the appropriate numbers on Your SHINE Protocol Worksheet (see Appendix C, page 275). When you are done reading the book, you will then have a treatment protocol tailored to your specific case. A fair number of treatments will be recommended. Each treatment will be marked by level of importance on the worksheet as a top, middle, or low priority. This way, you can choose how aggressively you want to proceed. For the medications I recommend, bring this worksheet to a holistic doctor and consult with him or her on how best to proceed. A large part of the protocol, however, can be done on your own naturally, without medications.

Once you are ready to begin your treatment, you can follow this basic timeline, adjusting as needed.

## WEEKS 1 THROUGH 3
Nutritional therapies, specifically multivitamin and ribose supplementation
Treatments for pain if needed
Sleep aids
Walk as comfortably able

## WEEKS 4 THROUGH 8
Hormonal therapies, continuing to use nutritional therapies and sleep aids

## WEEKS 9 THROUGH 20
Anti-infection treatments, adding one new treatment every one to three days, if necessary. Continue nutritional therapies, sleep aids, and hormonal therapies as needed. Begin to increase your walking, or increase the intensity of your exercise, as feels comfortable.

You should continue this regimen for six to nine months or until you begin to feel great for three months. Then slowly see if you can lower the dose of your treatments, without compromising how you feel. You may find that you do best continuing some treatments, especially the multivitamin and ribose supplementation, for the long term. In each chapter, I will discuss natural therapies first, as these are safer and often highly effective, and all that is usually needed for day-to-day fatigue. However, it is helpful to have prescriptions available as well, and these will also be discussed, usually as "intensive care" for CFS/FMS.

## IMPORTANT POINTS

Research has shown that more than 91 percent of people on the SHINE protocol report significant improvements.

1. *Sleep.* On average, most people do best with eight hours of sleep a night. For those with CFS/FMS, because your sleep center is not working, you need aggressive treatment to be sure that you can get at least eight hours of deep sleep each night.

2. *Hormonal support.* This includes treatment with bioidentical hormones for thyroid, adrenal, and ovarian/testicular support—even if your blood tests (which are very unreliable) are normal.

3. *Infections.* If sinusitis or irritable bowel syndrome are present, candida needs to be treated. In those with CFS/FMS, because your immune system is working poorly, there are many infections present that need to be treated.

4. *Nutritional support.* Make nutritional support easy without taking handfuls of supplements throughout the day by taking the Energy Revitalization System vitamin powder and D-ribose powder (see chapter 7).

5. *Exercise as able to condition.* For some people with CFS/FMS, this may mean walking just a few hundred feet a day.

At the end of each chapter, fill out the relevant questionnaire. It will tell you which treatments to check off in Appendix C, "Your SHINE Treatment Worksheet." When you finish reading the book, you will have tailored a treatment protocol to your specific case.

Many of the treatments will be natural remedies that you can use on your own. To get the full benefit, apply the SHINE protocol with the help of a knowledgeable holistic health practitioner (see chapter 13).

# PART 2

# Restore Energy Production with the SHINE Protocol

Restoring optimal energy production and eliminating those things that drain your energy are critical to restoring your vitality. Your checklist for doing this is the acronym SHINE:

**S**leep
**H**ormonal deficiencies
**I**nfections
**N**utritional support
**E**xercise as able

For those of you with day-to-day fatigue, simple measures can tune up each of these five areas. For those of you with the severe energy crisis that makes up CFS/FMS, we will finish the discussion of each of these areas in the sections called "SHINE Intensive Care."

Sleep is where we recharge our batteries and restore immune function. It is also critical for tissue repair, and therefore the elimination of pain.

Hormonal control is also essential. For example, the thyroid acts like your body's gas pedal. If it is sluggish, you will simply not produce adequate energy.

Because of excess sugar and antibiotics, yeast overgrowth in the gut (candida) is very common—and much more toxic than vaginal yeast infections. Treating candida not only can help eliminate chronic fatigue but also will often eliminate other chronic conditions, such as sinusitis and spastic colon. Those with CFS/FMS will often have picked up numerous other "hitchhiker infections" because their immune system is not working properly.

Nutrition, of course, is the key to health and energy production. We will teach you how to get outstanding and optimized nutritional support—without taking handfuls of tablets for the rest of your life. We will also discuss a special energy nutrient that in our recent study increased energy an astounding average of 61 percent after three weeks!

Exercise is key to conditioning, as your body has a "use it or lose it" approach to efficiency. Special rules apply in CFS/FMS, however, where exercise can cause people to crash instead of condition.

At this point, you're ready to start filling out the SHINE Treatment Worksheet (see Appendix C). The next five chapters will guide you through the key steps so you can get from where you are to where you want to be: feeling great.

# 4.

# S—Sleep: The Foundation of Getting Well

One of the most effective ways to improve energy and mental clarity is to simply get your eight hours of sleep a night.

But is it really that simple? Like so many other things in life, the answer is simply yes . . . and no! Let's put things into perspective.

Until 130 years ago the average night's sleep in the United States was nine hours a night. Average! That means as many people got ten hours a night as eight. Going back further in time, to most of human history, anthropologists tell us that the average night's sleep was eleven hours. Most nights, when the sun went down it was dark, boring, and dangerous to be outside. So people went to sleep. Then they woke up with sunrise, an average of eleven hours later. Now we are down to an average of about six and three-quarters hours of sleep a night, compliments of lightbulbs, radio, TV, the Internet, Facebook, and so on. This means the average person has lost 30 percent of their sleep in the last century.

In addition to simply not having time to get your eight hours of sleep a night, you may also find that the stress of modern life is causing insomnia. In this chapter, I will teach you how to treat day-to-day insomnia with natural therapies and sleep hygiene, and then discuss sleep intensive care for those with CFS and FMS.

### • • •     WHY IS SLEEP SO IMPORTANT?     • • •

Beyond giving us energy, sleep has a number of critical functions. For example, sleep:

1. is when tissue repair occurs, which is why poor sleep causes pain.
2. is also critical for proper growth hormone production. Growth hormone has also been called the "fountain of youth hormone" and is associated with looking young as well as increasing muscle and decreasing fat.
3. has been shown to be critical for immune function.
4. is important for weight regulation because appetite-suppressing hormones such as leptin are produced during sleep. Studies have shown that poor sleep was associated with an average six-pound weight gain. In a study of 68,183 women, followed over sixteen years, those sleeping five or fewer hours per night had a 32 percent increased risk of gaining thirty-three pounds relative to those who slept seven hours per night.

So it pays to make time for your eight hours of shut-eye. Not only will you have more energy and less pain, but you'll lose weight and look younger as well!

# Finding Time for Sleep

With life going haywire, you may wonder where to even find that extra two hours to get the shut-eye you need. Here are some thoughts to make it easier.

## STEP 1—YOU'LL NEVER GET IT ALL DONE

Realize that you will never get it all done, no matter how fast you run. In fact, you may have noticed that the faster you run and more efficiently you do things, the more life puts on your plate. So here's a secret. If you slow down and take the time to sleep, you'll find that fewer things find their way to your to-do list, and a lot of things seem to simply drift away that you didn't really want to do anyway. Then you'll find getting your eight hours of sleep a night will make you more efficient and effective, and you'll be enjoying the things you do more. Which leads to step two.

## STEP 2—KEEP WHAT FEELS GOOD
## AND DITCH THE REST

Make a list of most of the things you spend time doing in life, both at home and at work. Put these in two columns. Column 1 contains the things that feel good to do, or at least feel better to do than not to do. In column 2 put those things you *think* you should do but that feel awful. These include things like many committee meetings, school meetings, and other things that you don't really like but think you *should* do. This has been called "shoulding on yourself," thinking

"I should do this, I should do that." Here's your chance to stop that. I am giving you doctor's orders to cut out the things in your life that don't feel good and won't leave you fired or arrested if you cut them loose. So tell the chairwoman of the "committee of a thousand ways to waste everybody's time" that you would love to help, but the doctor said absolutely no more commitments.

Column 2 can also include things like watching the news past the first five to ten minutes. As long as you enjoy it, watch it. But when it starts making you feel bad (for me that's about seven minutes, and for my wife about a minute and a half), turn it off.

Once you start making these lists, you will find it is fun to take more and more things and put them in column 2. Then start tendering your resignations (I am not talking about to the job that pays your bills—yet). When I first realized this, I resigned from almost ten committees within a week, and have never missed them for a second. In fact, I dropped every committee except for one that I loved, which was starting a new school. It's been great—and has freed up the time needed for me to get my eight hours of sleep a night!

So now that you've learned how to make the time for sleep, here's how to handle insomnia and poor sleep quality.

## The Basics: Good Sleep Hygiene

The following are some things to consider:

Consume little or no alcohol before bedtime (optional).

Do not consume any caffeine after 4 p.m.

Do not use your bed for problem solving or doing work. If you are in the habit of using your bed for doing work, it is best to change your work area to another area of the house. If it helps you to fall asleep, you can watch relaxing television (perhaps on a timer that turns the television off if you fall asleep while watching) or read a relaxing book in bed until you can no longer stay awake.

Take a hot bath before bed if it's cold outside.

Keep your room cool.

If your mind races because your brain thinks it is daytime when it is really nighttime, continually focus your thoughts on things that feel good and do not require much "thinking energy." If you find that you cannot help but continue to problem-solve, get out of bed and write down all your problems on a piece of paper until you can think of no more—then set them aside and go back to bed. Do this as often as you need to. It may be helpful to schedule thirty minutes of "worry time" early in the afternoon or evening when you can update a check-list of your concerns. In addition, the herbal mix Sleep Tonight can be very helpful in this situation (see page 53).

### • • • WHAT TO DO WITH YOUR TO-DO LIST • • •

We seem to think that we're responsible for making everything happen. That kind of stress and anxiety can make a good night's sleep difficult to come by. I certainly struggle with this and have adopted a simple strategy that works for me. You may find something similar to be useful as well. When I feel overcome by details, I list my problems and projects on the left side of a page, and what I eventually plan to do about them (if anything) in the middle of the page. I consider these two columns to be what I

*(continued)*

leave in the hands of God, the universe, or whatever you wish to call it. Every so often, I move a problem from the "universe's" columns over to a third ("my") column on the right side. The items in the third column are the one or two things that I want to work on right now. I am constantly amazed at how the things that I leave in the "universe's" hands progress (on their own) as quickly as the things that I've put in "my" column.

I also have a separate list for day-to-day errands. I put a star by those items that must get done soon. I do other items if and when I feel like it. It is helpful to remember that neither you nor anyone else will ever get everything done. Just do those things that feel good to do on any given day, even if it's nothing. It will usually feel good to do the things that really have to get done. When I was doing general hospital internal medicine, I never heard a dying patient bemoan not having worked enough or not having completed all the errands on his or her checklist.

If your partner snores, get a good pair of earplugs and use them. The wax plugs that mold to the shape of the ear are often the best ones. It may also be useful to have either a sound generator that makes nature sounds or, better yet, a tape that induces stage 4 sleep (more about this later). Spouses of people with sleep apnea or snoring often also have severely disturbed sleep. You may need to sleep in a separate bedroom (after tucking in or being tucked in by your partner) until you find a way to sleep soundly through the snoring.

If you frequently wake up to urinate during the night, do not drink a lot of fluids near bedtime. Many people have frequent waking during the night and think they are waking up because they have to urinate. This is usually not the case.

If you were to wake up your spouse when you woke up and asked, "Honey, is your bladder full?" he or she would moan, "Uh-huh," and roll over and go back to sleep. Unfortunately, some people have learned to get up and go to the bathroom when they wake up at night. The bladder is kind of like a baby—if you teach the baby to wake up to play in the middle of the night (that is, if you go to the bathroom frequently), pretty soon it will wake you up to play at night. There is a simple way to remedy this problem. If and when you wake up during the night and you notice your bladder is full, just talk to it (in your mind, so your spouse doesn't think you're nuts) and tell it, "Nighttime is for sleeping. We will go to the bathroom in the morning when it is time to wake up." Then roll over and go back to sleep. If you still have to urinate five minutes later, then you can go to the bathroom. Most of you will find that your bladder will happily go back to sleep, and when you wake up in the morning, you won't even have to urinate as badly as you did when you woke up in the middle of the night. So don't worry if you get up to pee once a night. But if it's more, retrain your bladder to sleep through the night.

Put the bedroom clock out of arm's reach and facing away from you so you can't see it. Frequently looking at the clock aggravates sleep problems and is frustrating.

Have a high-*protein* snack (one to two ounces) before bedtime. Hunger causes insomnia in all animals, and humans are no exception. In addition, low adrenal (see chapter 5) can cause low blood sugar during the night, which will wake you up between 2 a.m. and 4 a.m. A handful of nuts or a hard-boiled egg at bedtime can help. If this is the problem, you will know the first night or two that you have the bedtime snack, as you will sleep through the night without waking as often.

# Getting Started

For almost all of the treatments recommended, you will know most of the effects (both positive and negative) that the treatment is going to have by the next morning. In rare cases, some of these treatments have the opposite of their intended effect, activating you instead of putting you to sleep. If this happens, don't use that treatment.

## • • •  SIDE EFFECTS OF SLEEP AIDS  • • •

For all of the medications listed in this section, any side effects that you may notice will usually occur the same day that you take the medication. I have not seen any "fly now, pay later" side effects from prolonged use of nonaddictive sleep meds. The exception is that less than 1 percent of people who take Ambien for more than a year develop an unusual and severe depression, which dramatically resolves one to seven days after stopping the sleep medication. In these rare situations I simply take the person off Ambien. I have not seen Ambien worsen symptoms in patients with preexisting depression. I've also seen sleepwalking and sleep eating in approximately one patient per thousand. These side effects mostly occurred when the individuals were taking over 10 milligrams a night.

I tend to be highly opinionated and very picky about what I find works well and what does not work as well. Because there is so much marketing out there for both natural and prescription remedies, it is hard for most nonexperts to tell what works. I decided more than twenty-five years ago that my position would be that of a patient advocate and that I work for you. Because of this, to maintain both credibility and objectivity, I accept no money from either pharmaceutical or natural products companies and direct that all royalties for products that I design be donated to charity.

# Natural Sleep Remedies

Most of the natural sleep remedies discussed here are not sedating, yet they help you fall asleep and stay in deep sleep. The good news is that many natural remedies that are effective for sleep also directly help pain because they are muscle relaxants. The first six herbs listed below are available in an excellent combination formula.

## MY FAVORITE NATURAL SLEEP AIDS

### Suntheanine
Theanine, an amino acid (protein) that comes from green tea, has been shown not only to improve deep sleep but also to help people maintain a calm alertness during the day.

Take 50 to 200 milligrams at bedtime, although you can also use it several times a day for anxiety.

## Wild Lettuce

Traditionally, wild lettuce has been found to be effective for anxiety and insomnia, as well as for headache, muscle pain, and joint pain. Wild lettuce may also decrease restless leg syndrome.

Take 30 to 120 milligrams at bedtime.

## Jamaican Dogwood

This extract acts as a muscle relaxant and also helps people to fall asleep while calming them. According to tradition, Jamaican dogwood was once used by Jamaican fishermen. Large amounts were thrown in the water. The fish would then fall asleep and be easy to net.

Take 12 to 48 milligrams of the extract at bedtime.

## Hops

The hops plant is a member of the hemp family, and the female flowers are used in beer making. It is not only the alcohol that lets college students fall down the steps when drunk without hurting themselves after a "kegger" party. It's also the hops.

Take 30 to 120 milligrams of a hops extract at bedtime.

## Passionflower (Passiflora)

This herb is commonly used throughout South America as a calming agent, even present as an ingredient in sodas. Passionflower has other pain-management benefits. In one animal study, it was shown that it decreases morphine tolerance, so that less medication is needed.

Take 90 to 360 milligrams of the extract at bedtime.

## Valerian

Commonly used as a sleep remedy for insomnia, valerian has many benefits, as shown in a number of studies, including an improvement in deep sleep, speed of falling asleep, and quality of sleep without next-day sedation. The benefits were most pronounced when people used valerian for extended periods of time, as opposed to simply taking it for one night.

Clinical experience shows that for around 5 percent of people, valerian is energizing and may keep them up. If this happens to you, you can use valerian during the day instead of at night, as valerian does have a calming effect and can be used during the day for anxiety as well.

Take 200 to 800 milligrams of the extract at bedtime.

To keep it simple, all six of these herbs can be found in combination in the Revitalizing Sleep Formula by Enzymatic Therapy. The dose is two to four capsules at bedtime if you just need them to help you stay asleep or one to two hours before bedtime to also help you fall asleep. They can also be used during the day for anxiety and pain.

I begin most of my patients who have insomnia on the Revitalizing Sleep Formula plus ½ to 1 milligram of melatonin. If they have trouble with their mind being wide awake at bedtime, this may suggest that their adrenal cortisol "stress hormone" levels may be too high at bedtime, despite being too low during the day. This is discussed in more detail in chapter 5 on hormones. In these cases I also have the person take one to two capsules of either Sleep Tonight by Enzymatic Therapy or Cortisol Manager by Integrative Therapeutics.

Both of these include a mix of phosphatidylserine, ashwagandha, and other natural compounds that help lower an elevated cortisol at bedtime. If this helps, you'll know within a few days. It is also a good idea to have a one- or two-ounce protein snack at bedtime (as discussed above) to keep blood sugar from dropping too low during the night.

Other natural remedies that help sleep include:

*Magnesium.* Taking 75 to 200 milligrams of magnesium at night is a good idea because it can help you sleep. Lower the dose if it causes diarrhea. A hot bath with one to two cups of Epsom salts will also raise magnesium levels while helping sleep.

*Lavender.* The smell of lavender can help sleep, as can lavender in capsule form. Simply put a drop of lavender oil on your upper lip or a few sprays on your pillow before bedtime. In addition, a new lavender capsule called Calm Aid by Nature's Way can help both sleep and anxiety.

*Lemon balm.* Lemon balm makes it easier to fall and stay asleep. Try 80 to 160 milligrams of lemon balm (also known as melissa).

*5-Hydroxy-L-Tryptophan (5-HTP).* Your body uses 5-HTP to make serotonin, a happiness molecule neurotransmitter that helps improve the quality of sleep. It also can help pain, stiffness, and anxiety and can even help some people lose weight. The dose is 200 to 400 milligrams at night. If taking other serotonin medications, use only with your holistic health practitioner's okay. It takes six to twelve weeks to see the full benefits of the 5-HTP.

*Delta-wave sleep-inducing compact discs or cassettes (look for Delta Sleep System CD by Dr. Jeffrey Thompson).* To fall asleep and stay in deep sleep, you can play the tapes or CDs and they will help your brain waves attune to and stay in the deep delta-wave frequency of deep sleep. If you wake up during the night, you can push your sound system's replay button. Better yet, get a CD or tape player that can replay continuously throughout the night.

## Other Important Sleep-Related Disorders

In addition to poor sleep caused by stress or hypothalamic dysfunction, let's look at two other common sleep problems, sleep apnea and restless leg syndrome (RLS).

### SLEEP APNEA

Sleep apnea is a condition in which you repeatedly stop breathing during the night. There are two main types of sleep apnea. One is obstructive, in which the pipe that carries air into the lungs gets blocked intermittently; the other is central, which means that the brain trigger that controls breathing stops working intermittently. Obstructive sleep apnea (OSA) is the condition that is most common.

In OSA, the pharynx (throat) repeatedly collapses during sleep. The person with OSA fights to breathe against a blocked airway, resulting in a drop in blood oxygen levels. Eventually, the sense of suffocation wakes the person, the throat muscles contract, the airway opens, and air rushes in under high pressure. When the airway is opened, the rushing air allows the patient to once again drift back to sleep, but it creates a loud, gasping sound. People with OSA are generally not aware that this is happening, although their bed partners often have severely disrupted sleep from the snoring and gasping. This cycle repeats itself many times throughout the night, and this constant waking from deep sleep, as well as the loss of oxygen in the blood, can cause next-day sleepiness, brain fog, poor concentration, and mood changes. Another side effect of OSA is high blood pressure. I generally recommend that anyone who has high blood pressure, snores, falls asleep easily during the day (especially while driving), has a shirt collar size of 17 inches or larger, or is overweight consider testing for sleep apnea. The screening test is best done at home, so ask your physician if it can be arranged that way. If it needs to be done in a sleep lab, ask them to do a "split night study" where they look for sleep apnea during the first half of the night and, if needed, check the CPAP (continuous positive airway pressure) measurements during the second half of the night. This way, it can all be done in one night instead of two. You'll be glad you did.

Although some doctors do not consider OSA to be significant until there are fifteen or more apneic episodes per hour of sleep, evidence suggests that even five or more episodes per hour are associated with increased risk of auto accidents and high blood pressure. Basically, if you tend to fall asleep easily during the day, the sleep apnea is likely to be significant.

For sleep testing, the lab will often recommend that you be off all sleep medications for several nights before doing the test. If you have not yet started sleep medications, this is reasonable. However, I recommend that patients who have been on sleep medications stay on them during the test because most CFS/FMS patients need the sleep medications, and as a doctor I need to know whether they are developing sleep apnea from the medication.

## THE POOR MAN'S SLEEP STUDY

Doing a sleep study (called a polysomnogram) in the sleep lab can cost upward of $2,000—and sometimes your insurance company will make your life miserable trying to get them to pay for it. Be sure to have them preauthorize the test. The diagnoses fatigue, daytime somnolence, snoring, and high blood pressure should be enough to get them to cover the study.

Another alternative? Set up a video camera at the foot of your bed to record yourself while you're sleeping. Position it so that you can see both your feet and your face. Then hit record, and go to bed with only a sheet on (you'll pull the blanket on later when you're sleeping, so don't worry). The next day, watch the tape. Do you have periods where you snore and stop breathing? If yes, is it only when you're lying on your back, or does it occur in any position? About how many times during the hour does it happen? If more than a few times during the hour, get the sleep study done doing a "split night study." Also check to see if your legs are jumpy and if it seems like this leg jumpiness seems to disturb your sleep. If yes, ask your physician to treat for restless leg syndrome (see below).

In addition, watching the tape is a good way to help you fall asleep!

## Causes of Sleep Apnea

The main cause of sleep apnea is being overweight. Just as fat deposits develop elsewhere in the body, they also occur in the tissue surrounding the throat. When lying down, the angle of the head can actually cause compression of the pipe that carries air into the lungs. As noted above, because of the often large weight gain caused by the metabolic disturbances in CFS/FMS, sleep apnea can occur and complicate treatment of these illnesses.

## Treating Sleep Apnea

The standard medical treatment for sleep apnea is to wear a CPAP (continuous positive airway pressure) mask over your nose or face while sleeping. This keeps a mild increased pressure in your throat, which keeps your airway from closing down. It is like a balloon where the neck of the balloon may close if you pinch it on both sides. But if you keep blowing into the mouth of the balloon, you can keep the balloon's neck open. During the sleep study, they do a CPAP titration. This is where they see how much pressure is needed in the mask to keep your sleep apnea from happening. CPAP is an excellent treatment for sleep apnea and is very helpful.

Many people are not willing to continue with the CPAP treatment because of the noise of the machine, the discomfort of wearing the mask, and the cost. However, patients who are able to tolerate the CPAP for at least three to six months become adapted to the treatment and eventually stop taking off their CPAP masks and throwing them across the room in the middle of the night. Fortunately, the newer CPAP machines have become much more user-friendly and better tolerated. Be sure to get one that also has a humidifier; otherwise it can dry out your mouth and lungs.

## THE TENNIS BALL CURE
## FOR SLEEP APNEA

Avoid sleeping on your back if the videotape shows that this is usually the position where you snore and have sleep apnea. Do this by taking a tennis ball, putting it into a cloth pocket, and then sewing it into the midback of your pajama shirt or a tight T-shirt. The tennis ball makes lying on your back uncomfortable, forcing you to roll onto your side or stomach without waking you. This works a lot better than having your spouse repeatedly jab you in the side during the night.

## RESTLESS LEG SYNDROME AND
## PERIODIC LEG MOVEMENT DISORDER

People with restless leg syndrome (RLS) have the sensation that they need to continually move their legs. When that happens predominantly at night, it is called periodic leg movement disorder of sleep (PLMD). Most people are talking about PLMD when they talk about restless leg syndrome.

It is not uncommon for your bed partner to be aware that your legs are kicking much of the night or are constantly moving. You may or may not be aware of your own movements. It has been estimated that as many as one-third or more of fibromyalgia patients have RLS/PLMD. Although the cause of RLS is not clear, experts suspect it comes from a deficiency of the brain chemical dopamine (called a neurotransmitter). It can also be aggravated by iron deficiency (having blood ferritin levels less than 60), nerve injuries, vitamin $B_{12}$ and folic acid deficiency, hypothyroidism, and other problems. In some people, RLS may be associated with the drops in blood sugar during the night (from adrenal fatigue—see chapter 5). Some medications, especially Elavil, can also aggravate RLS.

## Diagnosing RLS/PLMD

If you tend to scatter your sheets and blankets, and especially if you tend to kick your bed partner or if you note that your legs tend to feel jumpy and uncomfortable at rest at night, you probably have RLS/PLMD. You can also have a sleep study done to look for periodic leg movements. In real life, I do not waste $2,000 of the person's money to do a sleep study, as the history usually gives enough information, and nighttime videotaping is adequate confirmation. This is especially so because the treatments that would be used also help sleep and CFS/FMS, whether or not you have RLS/PLMD.

## Treating RLS

There are both natural and prescription approaches to treating RLS. Following are summaries of those that have been found to be most successful.

## Natural Treatments

Natural remedies focus on diet and nutritional supplementation. Avoiding caffeine helps, as does a high-protein snack at bedtime, which can decrease the tendency to have a drop in blood sugar (a drop in blood sugar can aggravate RLS).

The most critical treatment? Bringing your ferritin blood test (which measures iron stores) over 60 ng/ml. Technically, ferritin levels are considered to be in the normal range if they are over 12. This is insane, as considering a level over 12 to be normal will misdiagnose approximately 90 percent of people who have severe iron deficiency as being healthy and normal. But this is how it's done in today's medicine (see page 74—the problem with blood testing). I recommend taking an iron supplement that has 30 to 60 milligrams of iron and 100 milligrams of vitamin C, which helps the iron to be absorbed. Take iron supplements on an empty stomach, and if it causes upset stomach or constipation, it's okay to take it every other day. It is normal for iron supplements to turn your stool black. Aim to get your ferritin level to over 60 but under 120 ng/ml.

## Prescription Treatments

The medications Ambien, Klonopin (clonazepam), and Neurontin usually do a superb job in suppressing RLS, especially once the ferritin level is optimized. I tell patients to adjust the dose not only to get adequate sleep but also to keep the bedcovers in place and to avoid kicking their partners. As Klonopin is addictive (like Valium), I am more likely to use the other medications. Klonopin does have the added benefit of helping pain, so there are times that it may be helpful.

Although it is heavily marketed, I rarely use Requip. I find the other medications to be more effective and to have fewer side effects, while being low cost.

## FAST HEART RATE? YOUR SEROTONIN MIGHT BE TOO HIGH

The one caution I would note with 5-HTP is that if you are taking a number of treatments that increase serotonin (these include antidepressants like Prozac, Saint-John's-wort, Ultram, Desyrel, and the like), taking doses higher than 200 milligrams of 5-HTP can result in serotonergic syndrome, a life-threatening reaction caused by a too-high level of serotonin. Because of this, discuss the use of 5-HTP with your holistic doctor. This is a rare problem, however, and I have never seen a serious reaction myself. If you are taking any serotonin-raising treatments, though, it is reasonable to limit the 5-HTP to 200 milligrams at night.

Mild serotonergic syndrome can more often be associated with a constant fast heart rate, which is commonly seen as part of CFS and fibromyalgia. But when it gets more severe and potentially dangerous, it can be associated with a fever and feels like "the panic attack from hell." For anyone whose heart rate is constantly above 90, even if you are not taking 5-HTP, it is worth considering whether you are on too many treatments that raise serotonin and discussing *lowering* these with your doctor (if stopped suddenly, you may go through withdrawal). If the rapid heart rate is coming from these treatments, it should come down within a few days of lowering the dose. More often, though, in CFS/FMS the fast heart rate is from the autonomic dysfunction discussed on page 82, NMH and POTS.

# Sleep Intensive Care
# for CFS and Fibromyalgia

The most effective way to eliminate fatigue and pain in CFS/FMS is to get eight to nine hours of solid, deep sleep each night on a regular basis. In fact, disordered sleep is, in my opinion, one of the key underlying processes that drive CFS/FMS. Usually, when I lecture, I ask, "How many of you who have CFS/FMS can get at least seven to nine hours of solid sleep a night without medications?" Generally, out of three hundred to four hundred people in the audience, only one or two people, if any, raise their hands. When I speak with these people later, I usually find that they have sleep apnea, narcolepsy, or another treatable cause for their fatigue besides CFS/FMS.

Basically, if you can get a good night's sleep without taking anything, the probability is that you don't have CFS or fibromyalgia. This doesn't mean that the SHINE protocol won't help you; in fact, it helps many types of fatigue. It simply means that you have not blown a fuse and likely don't have CFS/FMS. This is why I teach doctors that the first thing to ask when people complain about fatigue and widespread pain is, "Can you get a good night's sleep?"

Why is this so? Because the hypothalamic circuit that goes off-line in CFS and fibromyalgia controls sleep. That's why asking about insomnia separates out CFS/FMS from other conditions so well.

If you follow the suggestions above, you can be sure that poor sleep hygiene is not your problem. This is important because your doctor may want to blame your insomnia on poor sleep hygiene. It is important to let him or her know that your problem is not poor sleep hygiene; it is hypothalamic sleep-center malfunction.

The hypothalamic sleep disorder in CFS/FMS is usually too severe to be dealt with by any single prescription or natural remedy. What works best is to mix these until you find a combination that gives you eight to nine hours of solid sleep a night without a hangover.

Whatever treatments you use, though, it is important that they not only increase the duration of sleep but also maintain or improve the deep stages (stages 3 and 4) of sleep. Unfortunately, many sleeping pills in common use—for example, Dalmane, Halcion, and Valium—actually worsen deep sleep. You want to be certain that the treatments and medications you use leave you feeling better the next day, not worse. In addition, long-term use of these addictive Valium family medications, and possibly even Ambien, may be associated with risks that are not seen with the other sleep aids we discuss.

There are several approaches to using sleep treatments in CFS/FMS. Some doctors prefer to use a single medication or treatment and push it up to its maximum dose. If that works, great; if not, they stop that medication and switch to another. Other doctors prefer to use low doses of many different treatments together until the patient is getting good, solid sleep regularly. I *strongly* prefer the latter approach in CFS/FMS, for two main reasons. First, my experience is that people with CFS and fibromyalgia can be *very* medication-sensitive, especially if high doses are used. Most of a medication's benefits occur at low doses and most of the side effects occur at high doses. Second, each medication is cleared out of the body on its own schedule, regardless of whether it is taken with other medications. If you take a low dose of a sleep medication, so that it is out of your body when it is time to wake up eight hours later, the blood level may not be high enough to keep you asleep all night. If you increase the dose to the level at which it does keep you asleep all night, it may not be cleared out of your body until 2 p.m. the next day, leaving you feeling very hungover. If, however, you combine low doses of four or five different sleep aids, each of them will be cleared out of your body by morning. Meanwhile, the effective blood levels that you have during the middle of the night from each treatment are additive and will keep you asleep. Because of this, most people with CFS/FMS find that they do best taking low doses of anywhere from three to seven different treatments, combining them to get eight to nine hours of solid sleep each night.

## BABY YOURSELF DURING STRESS— SO YOU SLEEP LIKE A BABY

It is not uncommon to see your sleep worsen again during periods of increased stress—whether physical or emotional—and the flaring of your illness. During these times, increase the treatments as needed to maintain at least seven to eight hours of solid sleep without waking prematurely or being hungover. I find that patients do not have a problem with continually having to escalate the dose, so I don't worry about increasing the treatments during periods of stress or flaring of your illness.

The best way to need less medication in the long run is to use as much as it takes to get eight hours of solid sleep each night for six months. When you are sleeping well and feeling better for six months, you can then start to start to reduce the treatments, as long as you continue to get eight hours of solid sleep each night. Many people find that they can taper off most sleep treatments after about eighteen months. Other people need to take some of the sleep treatments for years. This is okay. Either way, I suggest staying on something for sleep for the long term to decrease the risk of your CFS/FMS coming back. This could simply be the herbal remedy or a small dose of a sleep medication.

## Helpful Prescription Medications

There are dozens of medications that can help sleep in fibromyalgia. Below are my five favorites. Do not drive or operate hazardous equipment if you are sedated from the medications. Also, as with almost any medication and most herbs, do not get pregnant during treatment.

As we've discussed earlier, CFS/FMS patients usually do better with combining low doses of several medications than with a high dose of just one.

With hypothalamic sleep-center dysfunction, it is inappropriate to stop taking your sleep medications prematurely. Just as with high blood pressure, it is reasonable to stay on your sleep medications for years, if needed. Fortunately, after people are feeling better for six months, they usually find that they can lower the dose of sleep medication as the sleep center (in the hypothalamus) recovers. Keep in mind that if you use adequate medication to get eight to nine hours of solid sleep a night for six to nine months, you will likely need less sleep medication in the long run.

Let's look at the prescription sleep medications that work best in CFS/FMS:

*Zolpidem (Ambien).* This is my first choice of sleep medication for treatment in CFS/FMS because it is usually effective and well tolerated. It is also uniquely effective at helping people fall asleep, while the other medications help people stay asleep. Because Ambien is short acting (that is, it is out of your body after six hours), it is less likely to cause side effects than many other medications, but it also may not keep you asleep all the way through the night. A dose of 5 to 10 milligrams will likely give you at least four to six hours of good, solid sleep as a foundation. Doses of 10 milligrams or less are also less likely to cause addictive issues than higher doses.

If my patients wake up in the middle of the night, I have them simply keep half of a 5-milligram tablet by their bedside. When they wake during the night (as long as they have at least four hours before they need to drive), they simply bite on the tablet to crush it and put it under their tongue. Then they roll over and go back to sleep. It gets absorbed very quickly under their tongue, so it works quickly.

It is common to see severe rebound insomnia for about a week when you stop using this medication—that is, the need to use something else to assist your sleep. Because of this need for sleep assistance, if you have taken Ambien for more than two months, when you stop it, your doctor will likely need to prescribe some of the other medications or natural sleep remedies discussed in this chapter for a week or so to assist sleep during the adjustment period. In my experience, Ambien can also be helpful for restless leg syndrome. I do prefer to keep the total dose under 10 milligrams a night to avoid both addiction and problems with memory.

> ### • • •   A THOUGHT ON COSTS   • • •
>
> Generic Ambien costs about 10 cents a pill versus $3 to $4 for the brand name—and works every bit as well. This is the case for most medications when generics are available. Although there are unusual cases where the brand name works better, usually the price difference just reflects drug company profits. Personally and for my family, I go with the generic options when available.

*Trazodone (Desyrel).* Desyrel is marketed as an antidepressant (at a dose of 300 to 450 milligrams a day), but its main use in CFS/FMS is to treat disordered sleep. A dose of 25 to 50 milligrams is usually optimal for sleep.

*Gabapentin (Neurontin). Other related medications include tiagabine (Gabitril), or pregabalin (Lyrica).* These three medications are chemically related to gamma-aminobutyric acid (GABA), though their mode of action is more complex. Although the three are related, one will often work and be well tolerated even if the others are not. They are all effective for pain and restless leg syndrome and can markedly improve deep sleep. The main side effects are sedation, dizziness, and gastric upset. Lyrica may also cause weight gain at doses of 450 milligrams or higher. These are also discussed in chapter 9, "Natural and Prescription Pain Relief." Take 100 to 600 milligrams of Neurontin, 2 milligrams of Gabitril, or 50 to 300 milligrams of Lyrica at bedtime. I generally begin with Neurontin followed by Lyrica.

*Cyclobenzaprine (Flexeril).* This medication is a muscle relaxant and can be helpful for people who experience severe muscle pain with fibromyalgia. Interestingly, although the standard dose is 10 milligrams three times a day, studies show that just 3 milligrams at bedtime can be very effective in fibromyalgia for both sleep and lessening of next-day pain—with minimal side effects.

---

### • • •     CUDDLE YOURSELF     • • •

*Cuddle Ewe mattress pad* (www.prohealth.com or 800-366-6056). Lying on this cushioning sheepskin pad can help relieve pain when it interferes with sleep. In addition, getting wool sheets and pillowcases has been associated with a marked decrease in pain (especially when combined with wool long underwear during the day when it is cold outside) because the wool keeps your muscles warm, while wicking away any moisture from sweating.

---

I adjust the mix of natural and prescription treatments to be sure people get at least seven to eight hours of sleep a night. Although most people with CFS/FMS will be sleeping like kittens with some combination of the above, the long version of *From Fatigued to Fantastic!* and chapter 10 both discuss many other sleep options as well.

## GETTING STARTED

1. Be sure your sleep hygiene is okay.
2. Add natural remedies.
   A. melatonin—½ to 1 milligram
   B. Revitalizing Sleep Formula—two to four capsules at bedtime
   C. If wide awake at bedtime, try the Sleep Tonight herbal mix
3. Add medications (usually in this order and with these starting doses).
   A. Zolpidem (Ambien)—5 to 10 milligrams a night (can use part sublingually if you wake in the middle of the night)
   B. Gabapentin (Neurontin)—100 to 600 milligrams. If not well tolerated, consider Lyrica (pregabalin)—50 to 300 milligrams at bedtime.
   C. Cyclobenzaprine (Flexeril)—5 milligrams, ½ to one tablet at bedtime
   D. Trazodone (Desyrel)—25 to 50 milligrams at bedtime

## Important Points

- Getting eight to nine hours of solid, deep sleep a night without premature waking or having a hangover is critical to getting well.
- Begin with natural sleep aids. I recommend Suntheanine, wild lettuce, Jamaican dogwood, hops, passionflower, and valerian. These can be found in combination in the Revitalizing Sleep Formula by Enzymatic Therapy.

- Because of the severity of the sleep disorder in CFS and fibromyalgia, most patients will need to add prescription medications for at least six to eighteen months. A low dose of several medications is more likely to be effective without next-day sedation than a high dose of one medication. Ambien, Desyrel, Neurontin, and Flexeril (low-dose) are the four best prescription sleep medications. Most regular sleeping pills make you feel worse by keeping you in light sleep.

- Take whatever combination of treatments you need to get your eight hours of solid sleep a night.

- Treat sleep disorders such as sleep apnea, narcolepsy, and restless leg syndrome (RLS) if they are present.

## Questionnaire

(Check off treatments in Appendix C, "Your SHINE Treatment Worksheet.")

### Disordered Sleep

_____ 1. Trouble falling and/or staying asleep? If yes, is it

      _____ A. Mild (If yes, check #9.)

      _____ B. Moderate (If yes, check # 9 and 10.)

      _____ C. Severe (If yes, check #9, 10, 11, and 14–17 as needed.)

_____ 2. Is your mind wide awake and racing at bedtime? (If yes, check #12.)

_____ 3. Do you wake between 2 a.m. and 4 a.m.? (If yes, check #13.)

## Restless Leg Syndrome

_____ 4. Do your legs jump a lot at night or are your blankets (or bed partner) kicked around a lot at night? If yes, add #9, 14, and/ or 17 until your legs are still at night. Also videotape yourself at night, looking for restless legs, and ask your doctor to order blood work to check your ferritin level. If the ferritin is under 60, check off #5.

## Sleep Apnea

_____ 5. Do you snore?

## If yes:

_____ A. Are you more than twenty pounds overweight?

_____ B. Do you have periods where you stop breathing?

_____ C. Do you have high blood pressure?

_____ D. Do you fall asleep easily during the day?

If yes to A, B, C, or D, do a sleep study or videotape yourself sleeping to look for sleep apnea.

# H–Hormonal Support: Optimizing Adrenal, Thyroid, Testosterone, and Estrogen Function

Your body's metabolism is controlled by a series of glands that create chemical messengers called hormones. These hormones are controlled by feedback mechanisms in the hypothalamic master gland, which is the "circuit breaker" that malfunctions in CFS and fibromyalgia. Hormonal problems are also common in the general population, especially with the increasing number of chemicals and stress found in modern life. In CFS/FMS, hormonal problems are especially widespread.

## Functions of the Different Glands

The adrenal glands are really several glands in one. They are your body's key stress handler, while also helping balance your body's defense systems and maintaining blood pressure. If they are under-active, the result is fatigue, recurrent or persistent infections, hypoglycemia ("low blood sugar") with irritability and sugar craving, allergies or environmental sensitivities, low blood pressure, dizziness, and poor ability to cope with stress.

The thyroid gland is your body's gas pedal. It slows or speeds up the metabolism. If it is underactive, you can have fatigue, achiness, weight gain, poor mental functioning, and intolerance to cold.

The reproductive glands support and cycle the reproductive system. In women, if estrogen is low, you may feel worse around your periods and may feel depressed. If progesterone is low, the result is poor sleep and anxiety. In both men and women, low testosterone is a major contributor to pain, fatigue, and loss of libido.

Hormonal deficiencies often occur despite your hormonal blood tests being "normal." This chapter will present an overview of how to diagnose and handle these problems.

## The Problem with Blood Testing

Before we begin discussing each of the individual hormones, it is important to understand why we cannot rely on blood tests to tell us if there is a hormone-function problem. Many people with fatigue, and most people with CFS/FMS, have had the experience of going to the doctor convinced that their thyroid was low, only to experience the frustration of having the tests come back normal—often because the testing is not reliable.

Why is this happening?

By definition, the normal range for most blood tests is created by doing a large number of tests and defining only the highest and lowest 2.5 percent of the population as being abnormal (called "two standard deviations"). This does not work well if more than 2.5 percent of the population has a problem. To show how absurd it is to use a 2 percent cutoff, research has found that despite "normal" thyroid hormone levels, antibodies attacking the thyroid gland were present in 34 percent of FMS patients and as many as 19 percent of "healthy" controls. In addition, people whose thyroid tests were "normal" but in the low end of the normal range are a whopping 69 percent more likely to have a heart attack than those who are high normal.

One way to understand the difference between the "normal" range, based on two standard deviations (i.e., your not being in the lowest 2 percent of the population), and the optimal range, which you would maintain if you did not have CFS/FMS, is as follows:

Pretend your lab test uses two standard deviations to diagnose a "shoe problem." One hundred people go to the mall and their shoe sizes are measured. From these one hundred people, a normal shoe size range of 5 to 13 is established. As far as the shoe doctor is concerned, they could randomly give you any shoe between size 5 and size 13, and they would consider it totally normal for you—no matter what size your foot *is*! Of course, you would insist that the shoes did not fit because they didn't feel right on your feet. And the physician would then imply to you that you're crazy—because the shoe's size is in the normal range!

Sound familiar?

Like shoes, hormone levels are not "one size fits all." Because of this, treatment needs to be based predominantly on symptoms, using the blood tests only as one more piece of information. The goal is to restore *optimal* function while keeping lab results in the normal range for safety. Using this information, let's look at each gland and determine how to tell if there is a malfunction and how to optimize function. Let's begin with the adrenal gland—your "stress handler."

## The Adrenal Glands

The adrenal glands, which sit on top of the kidneys, are actually two different glands in one. The center of the gland makes epinephrine (also known as adrenaline, for the adrenaline "junkies" out there) and is under the control of the autonomic nervous system. Malfunction of the inner adrenal contributes to such symptoms as hot and cold sweats, neurally mediated hypotension (NMH), POTS (postural orthostatic tachycardia syndrome), and panic attacks.

The outer part of the adrenal gland, called the adrenal cortex, makes hormones that allow you to handle stress, regulate immune function, and maintain your blood pressure. Two key hormones are:

* *Cortisol.* The adrenal glands increase their production of cortisol in response to stress. Cortisol raises blood sugar and blood pressure levels and moderates immune function, in addition to playing numerous other roles. If the cortisol level is low, the person has fatigue, low blood pressure, hypoglycemia (low blood sugar) with irritability when hungry, poor immune function, an increased tendency to allergies and environmental sensitivity, and an inability to deal with stress. Sound familiar?
* *Dehydroepiandrosterone sulfate (DHEA-S).* Although what this hormone does is not clear, DHEA is the most abundant hormone produced by the adrenal cortex. If it is low, you will feel poorly. DHEA-S levels normally decline with age but appear to drop prematurely in CFS/FMS patients. Patients often feel much better when their DHEA-S levels are brought to the midnormal range for a twenty-nine-year-old.

# Symptoms of Adrenal Insufficiency

If your adrenal glands are underactive, what might you be experiencing? Low adrenal function can cause, among other symptoms:

- Fatigue
- Recurrent infections that take forever to go away
- "Crashing" during stress
- Hypoglycemia (low blood sugar with marked irritability when hungry)
- Low blood pressure and dizziness upon first standing

Hypoglycemia deserves special mention. To me, the single best test to tell if somebody needs adrenal support is to simply ask them if they get irritable when hungry. And we're not talking about day-to-day irritability but rather the "feed me now or I'll kill you!" type of irritability. If you're not sure if you have this, just ask the people around you.

People with adrenal fatigue have repeated episodes during the day where they become shaky and nervous, then dizzy, irritable, and fatigued. These people often feel better after they eat sweets, which improve their energy and mood for a short period of time. Because of this, these people often crave sugar. This makes their blood sugar level initially shoot back up to normal, which is what makes them feel better, but then makes it continue shooting up beyond normal. The body responds to this by driving the sugar level back down below normal again. The effect, mood- and energy-wise, is like a roller coaster. If you get super-irritable when hungry and you have to eat right away, adrenal support can be very helpful. A fringe benefit? It may also save your marriage or other relationships!

These episodes of low blood sugar occur because the adrenal glands' responsibilities include maintaining blood sugar during stress. Sugar is the only fuel that the brain can use. When a person's blood sugar level drops, he or she feels anxious, irritable, and then tired.

Don't bother doing the tests for low blood sugar or low adrenal, as these tests are geared to picking up the 1 in 100,000 people who have complete and life-threatening adrenal failure or insulin-producing tumors—not the problem we're looking at here.

## Problems with Adrenal Testing

Although the adrenal glands make several kinds of hormones, the lab tests for these glands use the production of cortisol as their marker. However, unlike other lab tests, where you are considered low if you're in the bottom 2 percent of the population, cortisol levels are only considered low when your adrenals have largely been destroyed and the condition becomes life-threatening—in other words, in approximately 1 out of 100,000 people. So it is either so low that they have to put you in the hospital and it can kill you, or it is considered totally healthy. At least this is the current medical viewpoint.

Let's look at this a bit more closely. Most people have morning cortisol levels of approximately 16 to 20 mcg/dl. However, a cortisol level of 10, half of what most people run, 8, or even 6.1 mcg/dl is considered *totally* normal. To technically have adrenal insufficiency, your morning cortisol needs to be less than 6 mcg/dl. Shockingly, adrenal insufficiency at a level of 5.9 mcg/dl is considered life-threatening. The method of evaluation goes from "normal" to deadly in just .01 mcg/dl. Unfortunately, I've seen an 8-mcg/dl variation on two cortisol levels accidentally done on the *same* tube of blood. So this rigid interpretation of test results doesn't make sense. Instead, if the fasting morning cortisol level is under 16 mcg/dl in CFS/FMS, *or* if symptoms suggest low adrenal, I consider a treatment trial of adrenal support.

# Why We Are Seeing More Adrenal Fatigue

If you think back to your biology classes in high school, you may remember something called the fight-or-flight response. This is a physical reaction that occurs during times of stress. During the Stone Age, when a caveman met an animal that wanted to eat him, the caveman's adrenal glands activated multiple systems in his body that prompted him to either fight or run. This reaction helped the caveman survive. In those days, however, people probably had a couple of weeks or months to recover before facing the next major stress.

In today's society, people often experience stress reactions every few minutes. For example, when driving to work, a woman is delayed because of heavy traffic. While sitting behind the wheel, she frets about the consequences of her walking into the office late. Every time she hits a red light or pulls up behind a car that has slowed down, her adrenal glands' fight-or-flight reaction goes off again.

Because of this, adrenal "stress handler" fatigue is very common—even in the overall healthy population. In CFS/FMS, it is even more common. In addition, I find low adrenal to be even more common in people whose CFS/FMS began with a severe flu-like illness.

## Treating Adrenal Insufficiency

Begin by cutting sugar and excess caffeine out of your diet; having frequent, small meals; and increasing your intake of protein while decreasing carbohydrates. It's best to cut way back on white flour and sugar and to substitute whole grains and vegetables. Fruit—not fruit juices, which contain concentrated sugar—can be eaten in moderation, so enjoy one to two pieces a day. If you get irritable, eat something with protein. For quick relief, put a quarter to half a teaspoon of sugar (a sugar packet is about one teaspoon) under your tongue and let it dissolve. This is enough to quickly raise your blood sugar level but not enough to put you on a sugar "roller-coaster ride."

Let's start by giving your adrenal glands the natural support that they need to heal.

## Natural Adrenal Support

Below are several things that can help your adrenal glands recover:

1. Adrenal glandulars supply the raw materials that your adrenal glands need to heal. It is critical, however, that you get them from reputable companies (I recommend Enzymatic Therapy and Standard Process for glandulars) so that the purity and po-

tency are guaranteed and so that you can be sure they come from cows that are not at risk of transmitting infections.

2. Vitamin C is crucial for adrenal and immune function. A dose of 500 milligrams is optimal.

3. Pantothenic acid, known as vitamin B$_5$, also supports adrenal function. Take 50 to 150 milligrams daily.

4. Licorice slows the breakdown of adrenal hormones in your body, helping to maintain optimal levels. There is no licorice in licorice candies in the United States because of this, as too much licorice can raise cortisol levels and blood pressure too high. Another beneficial effect of licorice is that it helps in the treatment of indigestion, and it is even as effective as the prescription heartburn medication Tagamet. Do not take licorice if you have high blood pressure, as too much licorice can cause excess adrenal function and worsen high blood pressure. You can safely take 200 to 400 milligrams a day of a licorice extract standardized to contain 5 percent glycyrrhizic acid.

5. Chromium also helps decrease the symptoms of low blood sugar. Take 200 to 400 micrograms a day.

If you'd rather not take these natural remedies separately, or just to simplify the supplementation, you can take Adrenal Stress End, which I helped the Enzymatic Therapy Company develop. Take one to two capsules in the morning. If symptoms recur in the afternoon, add another capsule at lunch. Adrenal Stress End, combined with the Energy Revitalization System vitamin powder, supplies everything noted above, as well as many other nutrients that will help support optimal adrenal function.

# Adrenal Intensive Care for CFS/FMS Neurally Mediated Hypotension and Postural Orthostatic Tachycardia Syndrome

If your blood pressure is low, you get dizzy upon standing, you crash after exercising, and you get a rapid pulse and a drop in blood pressure on standing, you might have neurally mediated hypotension (NMH) or postural orthostatic tachycardia syndrome (POTS). Often, NMH and POTS are simply labels given to some people with chronic fatigue syndrome. If so, adrenal support becomes especially important.

## ASSOCIATION BETWEEN POTS/NMH AND CFS

Unfortunately, when conventional doctors make a diagnosis of POTS or NMH, they typically don't recognize their association with CFS. A new study shows that they should.

Researchers at Vanderbilt University School of Medicine in Tennessee studied forty-seven patients with POTS. In POTS, when you stand up you have a speeding heartbeat and low blood pressure, causing symptoms like dizziness, nausea, and fatigue. Of these, 93 percent had severe fatigue with 64 percent were diagnosed with CFS. The folks with CFS had far worse cases of POTS than the others. "Fatigue and CFS-defining symptoms are common in POTS patients," concluded the researchers in an article published in *Clinical Science*.

But weak adrenal function isn't the only cause of POTS in CFS patients.

The area in your brain called the hypothalamus is a "circuit breaker" that controls energy for many key functions within your body, such as sleep and hormone production. It also controls blood pressure and heart rate through what is called the "autonomic nervous system"—a system that depends on healthy adrenal glands in order to function optimally. NMH and POTS are *disorders* of this autonomic function.

A diagnosis of POTS or NMH is likely to be a part of a larger CFS process if:

- ☐ Your fatigue is severe
- ☐ You have insomnia
- ☐ You're young (five to thirty years old)
- ☐ You tend to have a fast heart rate

One way to confirm this diagnosis is to undergo the "tilt-table test." In this test, you are strapped to a table and held upright to see if you pass out. Though it's the best diagnostic test for POTS/NMH, in my opinion it doesn't add much (except for expense and making you feel sick). I'm comfortable treating POTS/NMH in CFS patients on the basis of symptoms alone. In addition, see the "poor man's tilt-table test" discussed below.

The good news is that treating with the SHINE protocol can help not only CFS but POTS as well.

# Key Treatments for POTS/NMH

1. *Increase salt and water intake.* This supports the function of the adrenal glands.

2. *Get adrenal support—as discussed in this chapter.*

3. *Consider taking a stimulant such as Dexedrine, Adderall, or Ritalin.* I suspect these medications are overused in hyperactive kids but *underused* in CFS/FM patients with POTS/NMH. (Caution: Don't use more than 20 milligrams a day, as these drugs can become addictive at higher doses.)

4. *Consider taking ProAmatine (midodrine).* This medication can help maintain normal blood pressure. Over time, it may also help bring down a racing pulse.

5. *Consider taking Florinef.* This prescription synthetic adrenal hormone can help in POTS. Although more helpful in those under twenty years old, it may also be helpful in those with a chronically racing heart rate.

6. *Consider taking Prozac or Zoloft.* The class of antidepressant medications called SSRIs (selective serotonin reuptake inhibitors) is overused for depression (not a Prozac deficiency) but can help stabilize blood pressure. And studies show they help normalize the tilt-table test in POTS/NMH.

7. *Wear special support socks.* When you stand up, blood vessels in your legs contract, shooting blood back up to your head. In POTS, that doesn't happen as efficiently. Firm compression support socks (compared to mild compression socks, for varicose veins) can help those blood vessels do their job.

## A SIMPLE "POOR MAN'S TILT-TABLE TEST" FOR ORTHOSTATIC INTOLERANCE

Developed by Dr. David Bell, an excellent and very caring CFS researcher, this test is easily done in the office and requires only a blood pressure cuff—and a good nurse to catch the patient before the patient passes out.

The test is relatively simple.

- Check the blood pressure and pulse several times during a ten-minute interval while the person is lying down.
- Then have the person stand quietly (with a blood pressure cuff on) without moving or leaning on any object for thirty minutes, or as long as tolerated. Check the blood pressure and pulse every few minutes. If the person feels like he or she is about to faint, the test is stopped and considered a positive test.

This is called a poor man's tilt-table test, and Dr. Bell finds that most people with CFS flunk this test, showing one of the following three common abnormalities while standing:

1. A drop in systolic blood pressure (the top number) of more than 20 points.
2. POTS—the heart rate increases at least 26 beats per minute (bpm) over the resting heart rate.
3. Narrowing of the pulse pressure. The pulse pressure is the

(continued)

difference between the upper number of the BP and the lower number. For example, a normal person with a BP of 120/70 would have a pulse pressure of 50. It is actually this difference between the upper (systolic) and lower blood pressure numbers (diastolic) that circulates blood. If the pulse pressure drops below 18, it is abnormal, and not enough to help blood circulate properly to your brain and other tissues.

Patients should be tested in the late morning or early afternoon with no unusual activity prior to testing. Large meals and large volumes of fluid prior to testing should be avoided.

## Treating with Bioidentical Cortisol

More directly, and especially helpful in CFS/FMS, is treating the underactive adrenal problem with ultralow doses of adrenal hormone, which usually quickly banishes the symptoms of low blood sugar and can markedly improve energy. I like to begin with natural hydrocortisone such as Cortef (by prescription at most pharmacies) or, better yet, sustained-release hydrocortisone from a compounding pharmacy. I usually keep the dose under 15 milligrams of Cortef (hydrocortisone) a day. This immediately gives your body the support that your adrenal glands are unable to give, and may help you feel much better quickly. The added cortisol also takes some of the strain off your adrenals so that they can heal.

# Potential Toxicity of Cortisone

Adrenal hormones are essential for life. Without them, a person dies. But, as with any hormone, too much can be dangerous, and any cortisol supplementation should be closely monitored by your CFS/FMS specialist. In the early studies using adrenal hormones, the researchers had no idea what dose was normal and what was toxic. When they gave injections of the hormone to arthritis patients, the patients' arthritis went away and they felt better. However, they gave patients many times more than the normal amount, and many patients became toxic and died. Because of this, the researchers became frightened and avoided using adrenal hormones whenever possible. Medical students were taught to avoid adrenal hormones unless no other treatment choices existed.

The use of adrenal hormones needs to be put into perspective, however. Imagine if early thyroid researchers had given their patients fifty times the usual dose of thyroid hormone. Thyroid patients would have routinely died of heart attacks. The thyroid researchers, though, were fortunate enough to stumble upon the healthy dose early on and to skip negative outcomes (likely because too high a dose of thyroid caused immediate side effects). If they had not, people today would not be treated for an underactive thyroid until they were in a coma. Medical science is just beginning to learn that a person can feel horrible and function poorly even with a minimal to moderate hormone deficiency. Waiting for the person to "go off the deep end" of the test's normal scale is simply not healthy.

Fortunately, research has shown that the *very* low doses of cortisol we are recommending are safe. To put it in perspective, 5 milligrams of bioidentical hydrocortisone (Cortef) is approximately equal to 1 milligram of the synthetic prednisone, and I consider the bioidentical to be both safer and more effective unless one is treating inflammation. Unfortunately, most physicians are not familiar with the research on the safety of ultralow-dose hydrocortisone. This area is discussed at greater length in *From Fatigued to Fantastic!*

To summarize, if your CFS/FMS symptoms started suddenly after a viral infection, if you suffer from hypoglycemia (and irritability when hungry), or if you have recurrent infections that take a long time to resolve, you probably have underactive adrenal glands. About two-thirds of my severe CFS/FMS patients have underactive or marginally functioning adrenal glands or a decreased adrenal reserve.

Although I prefer natural products to pharmaceuticals, in this situation I am comfortable adding standardized bioidentical hormones to the natural therapies in those with CFS/FMS. This can markedly improve function and help your body to heal.

## Dehydroepiandrosterone (DHEA)

DHEA is another adrenal hormone that is often low. This hormone is checked with a DHEA-S blood level (not a DHEA level). If the level is under 90 mcg/dl in women or 300 mcg/dl in men, I add some DHEA. Though available without prescription, this hormone is best monitored by your holistic practitioner. Most women need 5 to 10 milligrams a day and men need 25 to 50 milligrams a day.

In women, half of their body's testosterone is made from adrenal DHEA, so taking DHEA can also correct low testosterone levels. But more is not better. If you have side effects, such as acne or darkening of facial hair in women, this suggests the DHEA dose is too high.

## POLYCYSTIC OVARIAN SYNDROME (PCOS)

We have also found that roughly 5 to 10 percent of women with CFS/FMS actually have elevated DHEA-S and testosterone levels. When I see this, I suspect and look for polycystic ovarian syndrome (PCOS) and insulin resistance. If a fasting morning insulin level is higher than 10 units/ml (suggestive of insulin resistance), especially if ovarian cysts or infertility are also present, these patients often improve significantly with a diabetes medication called metformin, 500 to 1,000 milligrams one to two times a day, which improves insulin sensitivity. This can also assist with restoring fertility, as well as helping the patient lose excess weight. As metformin can cause vitamin $B_{12}$ deficiency, it is critical that the vitamin powder be taken with it. Polycystic ovarian syndrome may also improve with low-dose hydrocortisone and with chromium supplementation of 1,000 micrograms daily.

## The Thyroid Gland

Thyroid problems are common in both day-to-day fatigue and CFS/FMS. Because of this, the discussion below applies to both.

The thyroid gland, located in the neck area, is the body's gas pedal. It regulates the body's metabolic speed. If the thyroid gland produces insufficient amounts of thyroid hormones, the metabolism decreases and the person gains weight. Other symptoms of hypothyroidism include intolerance to cold, fatigue, achiness, confusion, and constipation (though diarrhea from bowel infections is common in CFS/FMS).

The thyroid makes two primary hormones. They are:

- *Thyroxine (T$_4$)*. T$_4$ is the storage form of thyroid hormone. The body uses it to make triiodothyronine (T$_3$), the active form of thyroid hormone. Most synthetic thyroid medications, such as Synthroid and Levothroid, are pure T$_4$. These synthetics are fine if your body has the ability to properly turn them into T$_3$. Unfortunately, many people with CFS/FMS find that their bodies do not have this ability.
- *Triiodothyronine (T$_3$)*. T$_3$ is the active form of thyroid hormone.

There are many causes of low thyroid. In day-to-day fatigue, the main cause is low thyroid from autoimmune destruction of the thyroid gland (called Hashimoto's thyroiditis). In this autoimmune process, your body's immune system attacks and damages the thyroid. This can be diagnosed by a blood test called an "anti-TPO antibody." If the anti-TPO antibody is elevated, you likely have Hashimoto's thyroiditis (or another autoimmune thyroid disease) and may need to take thyroid supplementation for the rest of your life. This is one of the only thyroid blood tests that gives a straightforward and reliable "yes or no" answer.

In CFS/FMS, low thyroid can also come from hypothalamic dysfunction. In addition, research suggests that when CFS/FMS occurs, the body may not be able to adequately turn $T_4$ into $T_3$, or it may need much higher levels of $T_3$ (called thyroid receptor resistance). In all three of these situations, the standard blood tests may be totally normal despite the person desperately needing thyroid hormone.

## The Problem with Most Thyroid Tests

Put simply, most thyroid tests miss the vast majority of people with CFS/FMS who need thyroid hormone. The main blood test, called the TSH, is grossly unreliable in the presence of hypothalamic dysfunction. Meanwhile, having to be in the lowest 2 percent of the population for the actual level of the $T_4$ hormone (called the Free $T_4$) to get treatment is absurd. Meanwhile, we have no test that accurately measures $T_3$ function. So the problem with thyroid testing is that it is hopelessly unreliable—unless you understand what the normal ranges mean and interpret the tests in the context of the person's symptoms. So if somebody is tired, is achy, has unusual weight gain, or has cold intolerance, and has a thyroid Free $T_4$ test even in the lowest third of the population (not the lowest 2 percent), that person deserves a trial of thyroid hormone. Make sense? It's simple common sense!

## Treating an Underactive Thyroid

Though I use the guidelines above to decide when someone with day-to-day fatigue is given thyroid hormone, almost everybody with fibromyalgia deserves a treatment trial with thyroid unless their thyroid hormone (free $T_4$) is in the upper 25 percent of the normal range—at which point I look for an overactive thyroid.

We are constantly learning powerful new tricks for treating hypothyroidism, and there are many reasonable treatment approaches. In fact, like trying on shoes, it is not unusual for people to need to try several different thyroid protocols to see what works the best for them.

Here are the four most common approaches.

1. If the anti-TPO antibody test, which looks for your body's immune system accidentally attacking your own thyroid (most commonly, a form called Hashimoto's thyroiditis, which I described earlier), is normal, I begin with a prescription desiccated thyroid. This is simply ground-up thyroid gland. Although Armour thyroid used to be my favorite, the company reformulated it, and the new product worked poorly for many people. It has been redone again, and seems to be more effective, but it will take time to be sure. Because of this, it is reasonable to use Nature-Throid or Westhroid instead, although this is a bit harder to find at most pharmacies. Another option is to begin with desiccated thyroid made by a compounding pharmacy (see below), as a "gold-standard" to see what your body needs. Then you can switch to Armour or other desiccated products that may be covered by your insurance if they work equally well for you.

2. If the anti-TPO antibody test is positive, I am less likely to give thyroid glandulars out of a concern that the immune system might attack the proteins in those as well. In these cases, I am more likely

to simply give a combination of the $T_4$ and $T_3$ hormones without the glandular (also made by a compounding pharmacy).

3. If the thyroid forms above, which also contain active $T_3$, make people shaky or hyper, I am likely to simply use the plain $T_4$ (Synthroid) from a regular pharmacy.

## THYROID INTENSIVE CARE FOR CFS/FMS

If people with CFS or fibromyalgia do not respond to one of the above, especially if their reverse $T_3$ blood levels are high normal, I suspect that there may be what is called "thyroid receptor resistance," which is like the cells being "hard of hearing" to the thyroid hormone. In these cases, I consider an approach developed by the late and excellent doctors Broda Barnes and John Lowe. This involves giving a therapeutic trial of high-dose $T_3$ thyroid hormone, which is discussed in more detail in *From Fatigued to Fantastic!*, and needs to be given by a CFS/FMS specialist.

What treatment will work best often depends on what is causing your thyroid levels to be inadequate. Like trying on shoes, seeing what treatment *feels* best to you is much more reliable than trying to chase blood tests.

If you are shaky or hyper on thyroid, or have a racing heart (for example, a pulse over ninety beats per minute), lower the dose. Rapid pulse is common in people with CFS/FMS regardless of whether they're taking thyroid hormone, and if this is occurring, it may need to be treated before you can take thyroid (see POTS/NMH above). If taking Armour thyroid or $T_3$ hormone, splitting the dose to half in the morning and half at night, or switching to Synthroid, is less likely to cause you to feel hyper. Also, do not take thyroid hormone within six hours of taking iron or calcium supplements, or you won't absorb the thyroid.

Once you and your physician have found the form and dose of thyroid that feels best, your doctor should check the free $T_4$ blood level four to six weeks later to make sure it is in the normal range for safety. I recommend that people with CFS/FMS decline taking a TSH test to monitor thyroid dosing. It will be low (because of the hypothalamic dysfunction) and your doctor will incorrectly think you're on too much thyroid, even if your blood $T_4$ hormone levels are low normal. The TSH test can actually cause more harm than good, especially in fibromyalgia. Although many patients can stop taking thyroid hormone after twelve to twenty-four months, people can stay on desiccated thyroid or Synthroid for as long as it is needed. If on pure $T_3$ dosing of 35 micrograms or more, no blood testing is reliable and the dose is adjusted based on clinical symptoms.

All thyroid treatments must be prescribed and monitored by a physician. Holistic physicians are more likely to be familiar with optimizing thyroid support. Unfortunately, most other doctors are (incorrectly) trained to stop increasing the dosage of thyroid hormone once an individual's TSH thyroid tests in the "normal" range—even if the person's clinical signs and symptoms show that the dose is quite inadequate.

Synthetic $T_4$ (Synthroid) and pure $T_3$ (Cytomel) are available at any pharmacy. Sustained-release $T_3$, which works better for many patients, can be made by a compounding pharmacy. When you settle on an optimal dose, the compounding pharmacy can then make a single capsule of that dosage to be taken one or two times a day. This is less expensive because the cost tends to be based more on the number of capsules than the actual amount of $T_4$ or $T_3$ thyroid hormone in each capsule.

## Potential Side Effects

If someone has blockages in the arteries that feed the heart and is on the verge of a heart attack, taking thyroid hormone can trigger a heart attack or angina, just as exercise can. Thyroid treatment can trigger heart palpitations as well. These are usually benign, but if chest pain or increasing palpitations occur, stop the thyroid supplementation and call your doctor at once. Because of this concern, I may recommend that patients at significant risk of angina have an exercise treadmill test done before treatment, even if they can't complete the test.

To put the risk in perspective, of the many thousands of my patients taking a standard thyroid supplement, none experienced heart attacks or other major health issues from taking it. For the high-dose $T_3$ protocol, heart attacks, although quite rare, can be seen and I recommend those protocols only be used by physicians familiar with their administration. In the long run, research shows that thyroid treatment for subclinical hypothyroidism is *much more likely to decrease* one's risk of heart disease—by a whopping 39 percent!

## THE BEST THYROID SUPPORT GROUP LEADER IN THE WORLD!

For those of you looking for the most helpful, reliable, and up-to-date thyroid information available, I happily and strongly recommend Mary Shomon. Her Web site is www.thyroid-info.com, and you can sign up for her free e-mail newsletter while also accessing a wealth of other resources. More good news? She is now doing thyroid coaching, offering personal guidance for you and your physician on how to optimize *your* thyroid treatment.

# The Reproductive Glands—Menopause and "Manopause" (Andropause)

Many people going through midlife develop fatigue, poor libido, or depression. This includes men and women alike. Just as your car needs a tune-up when it hits 45,000 miles, so does your body.

Both research and clinical experience have found that if the estrogen and testosterone levels in females or the testosterone level in males is suboptimal, natural support, and often even a trial replacement using bioidentical hormones, can result in dramatic improvements.

# Male Menopause
## (Testosterone Deficiency)

Testosterone is practically synonymous with manhood. Unfortunately, testosterone levels in men often decline by the time they're in their midforties, producing symptoms such as fatigue, depression, loss of motivation, irritability, poor concentration, memory loss, aches and pains, and a host of other problems. The symptoms or signs that I consider to be suggestive for low testosterone in men include:

1. Loss of libido
2. Erectile dysfunction
3. A combination of high blood pressure and elevated cholesterol (which usually reflects what is called "metabolic syndrome")
4. Diabetes
5. CFS or fibromyalgia

If the testosterone level is in the lower 30 percent of the normal range, and the person has one or two of the symptoms above, I consider treatment with bioidentical testosterone creams. I'm especially likely to recommend the testosterone if deficiencies are contributing to health problems such as high blood pressure, high cholesterol, or diabetes. I generally do not recommend testosterone injections or oral testosterone.

## KNOW THE DIFFERENCE!

It is important that we not confuse giving safe levels of healthy *bioidentical* natural testosterone with the high-dose, synthetic, and toxic testosterone that can be misused in sports. The latter is what you will hear discussed as "steroids" in the news, and can be quite toxic.

# Treating Low Testosterone in Men

If your testosterone level is low, I recommend talking to a holistic doctor (see chapter 13). These practitioners specialize in giving men and women over forty-five years of age regular "tune-ups" to keep their health and vitality optimized. Basically, I think it is very helpful for males over forty-five years of age to get a solid tune-up—which includes more than simply testosterone. These are much different from the checkups people get at their family doctor's, which simply look for signs of disease, with little to no focus on optimizing energy and vitality.

For men under fifty years of age, it is often preferable to stimulate your body's own production of testosterone, using either a medication called clomiphene (25 milligrams) at bedtime each Monday, Wednesday, and Friday, or using other approaches such as HCG (human chorionic gonadotropin) hormone injections to stimulate your body's own natural hormone production. A clomiphene stimulation test can see what approach is best for a given individual. For those over fifty, I am more likely to recommend a topical bioidentical testosterone cream or gel, applying 25 to 75 milligrams to the skin daily.

You can get the testosterone cream by prescription (e.g., Fortesta) from a regular pharmacy. It is obscenely expensive but is often covered by prescription insurance.

The good news: you can also get prescription testosterone cream from a compounding pharmacy that creates customized medications on-site. A compounded version of the drug is *much* less expensive but just as effective. This is an excellent option for those without prescription insurance that covers testosterone.

(To find a compounding pharmacy, see Appendix E, "Other Resources.")

Caution: Wash your hands after applying the gel or cream to your skin. If you don't wash them, and then touch someone else—such as your spouse—she can develop a high, unsafe blood level of testosterone. This increases the risk of her getting diabetes. Some men think that it will raise their wife's libido. Unfortunately, it may be for another man! So it's best to apply the testosterone on your thighs or other areas that people don't touch so the cream does not get on anyone else. Rotate the area you put the cream on, or less may be absorbed over time.

Most men feel best with a blood level around the 70th percentile of normal range, and that's what I aim for in my patients, especially if it can be achieved with a dose no higher than 50 to 75 milligrams a day. Follow-up blood testing is best drawn two to three hours after applying the testosterone. Otherwise, the blood levels can be falsely low.

## • • • DON'T CHASE A TESTOSTERONE HIGH! • • •

Caution: Too high a dose can initially cause a bit of a "libido high," but your body adapts to the extra testosterone by increasing a type of protein that binds to testosterone and makes it inactive. Sometimes men then try to "chase the feeling" by pushing the dose higher and higher—not a good idea!

Over time, doctors who treat their patients with bioidentical hormones (including bioidentical testosterone) are finding that lower doses of bioidentical hormones may be more effective than higher doses. For testosterone, I now sometimes limit the dose to 50 to 75 milligrams a day—quite a bit lower than the 100-milligram doses used in the past. Once you're at the 50-milligram dose, if the blood level of testosterone is not too high (in which case the dose should be lowered), it's reasonable to stay at this dose and go no higher unless your symptoms require it.

Make sure your blood levels don't exceed the upper limit of normal, which can cause problems, such as acne. Fifty may be the new thirty, but I don't think you want to be a teenager again!

# Menopausal Problems

In women, estrogen and progesterone levels also start dropping in the midforties, but the blood tests will miss the deficiency for the first five to twelve years that your body is missing the estrogen! So once again, the tests are not reliable.

How do you know if bioidentical estrogen and progesterone may help you?

Although estrogen and progesterone deficiency can cause a host of problems, including fatigue, brain fog, headaches, and insomnia, these symptoms can also be caused by many other problems. They are more likely to be caused by low estrogen/progesterone if you also have:

1. Worsening of insomnia, fatigue, and headache around your period
2. Decreased vaginal lubrication
3. Loss of libido
4. Hot flashes

Remember, however, that menopause is not an illness, any more than puberty is. If you feel comfortable weathering the change, it's fine to simply ignore the symptoms or live with them. Unlike low testosterone in men, which can be associated with high cholesterol and hypertension and greater risk of heart disease, low estrogen or progesterone does not cause these problems in women.

The time to consider addressing perimenopause or menopausal symptoms is if they are uncomfortable. Some women also find that they feel and look younger on the bioidentical hormones, and prefer them for this reason as well.

But whether you prefer to simply add more edamame to your diet (as discussed below), take an herb, take bioidentical hormones, or simply weather the changes, it's always a personal preference that depends on you. There is no "right" or "wrong" answer for how to approach the natural process of menopause. Choose the options that feel best to you. As a woman, it is especially important to learn to trust your intuition/feelings and what your body is telling you.

## FIFTY CAN BE THE NEW THIRTY FOR WOMEN, TOO!

As you can tell, I strongly believe that both men and women deserve to get a major tune-up once they turn forty-five years of age. Just like your car would feel like it was on its last legs (or perhaps I should say tires) if it had never had a tune-up or oil change by the time it hit 45,000 miles, many people complain of symptoms they (or their physician) attribute to age by the time they hit forty-five. Most often, it is not age. Rather, you simply need a tune-up! This should address not only hormone deficiencies but also other factors such as optimizing bone density; addressing skin and hair health; and addressing sleep and many of the other factors discussed in this book.

These tune-ups are not the same as getting a physical. The purpose of the latter is to screen for illnesses, whereas the tune-up is to *optimize* function and vitality.

See one of the physician organization Web sites in chapter 13 to find a practitioner familiar with these concepts. You deserve to look and feel great!

# Therapeutic Options for Menopausal Problems

### EAT MORE EDAMAME

More commonly known as soybean pods, this tasty food is a standard appetizer in Japanese restaurants. You can find it in the frozen food section of most supermarkets and health food stores.

Edamame is rich in phytoestrogens, a weaker, plant-based version of estrogen. Eating a handful a day raises your estrogen levels naturally—the dietary approach traditionally used by Japanese women for centuries to manage menopause symptoms. (Eat the pea-like beans inside the pod, not the pod itself.)

## TAKE BLACK COHOSH FOR HOT FLASHES AND NIGHT SWEATS

Along with edamame, you may want to take the herb black cohosh, which my patients find very helpful. Black cohosh stabilizes the functioning of the autonomic nervous system, which can decrease hot flashes and night sweats.

I prefer Remifemin, from Enzymatic Therapy, a black cohosh product that has been proven effective in dozens of studies. Take two capsules two times daily for two months (it takes two months to see the full effect). After that, you can usually lower the dose to one capsule daily.

### NEW RESEARCH ON FISH OIL FOR MENOPAUSE

Although I would begin supporting your body through peri-menopause with edamame and Remifemin, if more support is needed, consider fish-oil essential fatty acids for hot flashes. Canadian researchers studied ninety-one women with hot

*(continued)*

flashes (an average of 2.8 hot flashes a day). Those given fish oil had an average decline of 1.6 hot flashes a day; there was an average decline of 0.5 in the placebo group. I recommend Vectomega by EuroPharma, one to two tablets a day.

# For Severe Menopausal Symptoms and CFS/FMS

## TAKING BIOIDENTICAL HORMONES

If symptoms of estrogen/progesterone deficiency are still problematic despite the above, especially in those with CFS/FMS, I consider bioidentical estrogens and progesterone to be healthy. These are not to be confused with synthetic or horse estrogens such as Premarin and conjugated estrogens, or synthetic progestins like Provera. I consider the synthetic hormones to be horribly toxic, in contrast to the bioidenticals, which I consider to be health promoting.

Using the bioidentical estrogen and progesterone is especially important:

1. In women who had a hysterectomy or had their ovaries removed before age forty-five, even if the ovaries are left in, a hysterectomy will routinely cause estrogen deficiency within two years. I have found that younger women are much less able to tolerate low estrogen than women in their fifties, and the younger women will need the bioidentical hormones.

2. In women with CFS/FMS, low estrogen and progesterone often are occurring because of the hypothalamic control center dysfunction, and not simply because of perimenopause.

The main treatment I use in my perimenopausal and menopausal patients is the bioidentical estrogen hormone Biest, along with natural progesterone.

These hormones are compounded into a skin cream by a compounding pharmacy. If vaginal dryness is an issue, asking the compounding pharmacy to make a cream for vaginal use can be very helpful. (See Appendix E, "Other Resources.")

As our understanding of the use of bioidentical hormones grows, many holistic physicians are finding that even very low doses can be effective, a plus for safety. Here are the details:

For many years, a common dose was 2.5 milligrams of Biest and 50 to 100 milligrams of progesterone daily. Clinical experience is suggesting that a tiny fraction of this dose may be even better. I currently recommend 0.1 to 0.5 milligrams of Biest a day (⅒ to ⅕ of the old dose), along with 30 milligrams of topical progesterone. In women already using higher doses, I slowly lower the dose, as feels comfortable to the patient. If they have adapted to the 2.5-milligram dose and feel best on that dose, that's okay, and I leave them on their current dose. If it does not leave you feeling poorly the week you are off the hormones, it is okay to not take the estrogen/progesterone the first week of each month.

So the good news? Women are not only using less to achieve the same results—they're spending less. The pharmaceutical companies have found that women prefer bioidentical hormones, so they are now available from your regular pharmacy, where they may be covered by insurance.

Simply use an estrogen patch, all of which now have bioidentical estradiol. Because only very low dosing is needed (⅒-milligram patch or lower), it's fine that the patch has only one of the two major estrogens found in Biest (though in the future, I hope they will combine both, including the estriol). In addition, bioidentical progesterone is available in the prescription Prometrium (100 milligrams at bedtime). This is equal to 30 milligrams of the topical cream.

More good news? Although the Women's Health Initiative (WHI) study raised the concern of breast cancer from using Premarin (the very strong and toxic horse estrogen Premarin) when started in women in their sixties, new research using the lower dose, starting at a younger age, or using more bioidentical estrogens is seeing *no* increased cancer risk. So women taking these hormones can feel much safer!

Again, it is important to remember that the hormone blood tests will stay normal until you are estrogen and progesterone deficient for five to twelve years. This is yet another example of where it is important to remember, "Treat the person, not the blood test."

## CONSIDER TESTOSTERONE, TOO

I've found that a deficiency of testosterone in women can cause some of the problems that occur with low levels of testosterone in middle-aged men: fatigue, depression, osteoporosis, weight gain, muscle achiness, and low libido.

As with men, I test for low free testosterone levels (not only total testosterone, which measures only the inactive, storage form of the hormone).

If levels are in the lower quarter of the normal range, I treat with a testosterone cream made by a compounding pharmacy. The usual dose is ½ to 1 milligram a day. (As with estrogen and progesterone, we are finding that lower doses than those used in the past are equally effective.) With this dosing, most menopausal women notice they have more energy, thicker hair, younger skin, and an improved libido. Testosterone supplementation is especially important in women with chronic pain, as both the pain and pain medications can cause testosterone deficiency, and testosterone deficiency (even with normal blood tests) will amplify pain.

If you also are taking estrogen and progesterone, the compounding pharmacy can combine the three hormones in one cream, for ease of application and lower cost. In addition, the hormones can be taken in a once-a-day capsule if the woman is not comfortable using the creams. If urine incontinence or decreased vaginal lubrication are present, get the cream made for vaginal application, and apply it in the vagina and to the inner lips of the labia (outer vagina). Many women find this works much better for overall health improvement than taking the estrogen by mouth or simply applying the cream to the skin.

## NARCOTICS CAUSE TESTOSTERONE DEFICIENCY

Chronic use of narcotic pain medications like Vicodin, codeine, and oxycodone will routinely cause testosterone deficiency in both men and women. Low testosterone equals increased pain. This cycle contributes to the need for ever-increasing doses of

*(continued)*

narcotics in some people. Because of this, any pain patient who needs chronic narcotic pain medications should have their testosterone levels kept at an *optimal* level—using only bioidentical testosterone. This not only decreases pain but also improves healing and overall well-being.

Optimizing testosterone levels can result in many benefits in people with CFS and fibromyalgia. Though it can take six to twelve months to see the full effects, sometimes people start improving in a few days to weeks. Here are benefits of optimizing testosterone levels.

1. In women with fibromyalgia, a study done by Professor Hillary White of Dartmouth University showed that giving natural testosterone decreased pain.
2. Fibromyalgia and CFS are associated with decreased red blood cell levels. In fact, most people with CFS/FMS are anemic despite having normal blood tests. Testosterone supplementation is a highly effective way of increasing the red blood cell levels.
3. Testosterone can improve libido, which is low in 73 percent of CFS and fibromyalgia patients.
4. Testosterone increases bone density, therefore decreasing the risk of osteoporosis.
5. Testosterone improves mood and decreases depression.
6. Testosterone increases muscle strength and decreases fat levels.
7. Low testosterone is associated with an increased risk of high cholesterol, angina, and diabetes in men.
8. Chronic fatigue syndrome has been associated with a possible

decrease in the heart's ability to pump blood, and testosterone improves heart function.

### • • • A FEW OTHER TREATMENT TIPS • • •

1. In women, simply optimizing DHEA hormone levels can often adequately increase testosterone levels. This will not help in men because men need much higher levels.
2. Acne suggests that the testosterone dose is too high, as does increased facial hair in women.
3. With hormone creams in general (for both men and women), rotate the skin area you apply it to; otherwise, absorption drops over time.
4. Wash your hands after putting on the estrogen. Apply it to an area where it won't rub off on your gentleman. I know you may want to bring out a bit of his understanding feminine side, but you don't want him growing breasts!

## Side Effects

The more common side effects of bioidentical estrogen and progesterone (as opposed to the very toxic synthetics, whose side effects could fill a book) are fluid retention, moodiness, spotting, and breast tenderness.

In those being treated for CFS/FMS, it is important to be aware that using the SHINE protocol will routinely result in your periods becoming irregular for six to twelve months—whether or not you take estrogen. This occurs in part because your hypothalamus cycles back to its normal rhythm as it starts to heal, and this controls the timing of your cycle.

## PREGNANCY AND CFS/FMS

Women often worry about getting pregnant with CFS/FMS. The good news is that most people with CFS/FMS do very well with pregnancy—and can do so even after the pregnancy, given the proper support.

Most of you will actually feel much better during your pregnancy. It is after the pregnancy that you'll need both nutritional and hormonal support to prevent the CFS/FMS from recurring. I do recommend that, if possible, you follow the treatment protocol discussed in this book for a year before getting pregnant, so you can stop the medications and other treatments that would not be appropriate during pregnancy, without losing the benefits. Although most people with CFS/FMS do not have problems with infertility, it is more common in this population than in the non-CFS/FMS population. The good news is that there are many effective natural treatments for infertility. Because they are not expensive, however, they do not get the attention that in vitro fertilization gets. (For more information on both natural treatments for infertility and how to have a healthy pregnancy, see www.vitality101.com.)

# Growth Hormone

Inadequate levels of growth hormone (GH) may be an important factor for some patients with CFS/FMS who do not respond to the rest of the SHINE protocol. It can be detected with a blood test called an IGF-1 level.

Because these injections are expensive and can have side effects (e.g., carpal tunnel syndrome), I prefer to have patients first do SHINE, as most people won't need these injections. The top three things that naturally increase your body's own production of GH are:

1. Sex
2. Exercise
3. Deep sleep

I happily recommend all three!

As you can see, many problems can occur when the body's glands do not function properly. The good news is that most can be effectively treated. In my experience, this often results in dramatic improvement.

# Important Points

- Hormonal deficiencies are becoming increasingly common in both the general population and CFS/FMS sufferers.

- Blood testing is not a reliable way to tell if you need hormonal support. The normal range for most blood tests does not tell you whether your hormone levels are adequate; rather, it measures only whether you are in the lowest 2.5 percent of the population.
- Tired, achy, weight gain, and cold intolerant? These suggests low thyroid regardless of the test results. If you get very irritable when hungry, consider adrenal support.
- Optimizing testosterone can be very helpful for both men and women over forty-five years of age or in those with chronic pain.
- Bioidentical estrogen and progesterone in women can be helpful, especially if symptoms of deficiency are worse around their period.

## Questionnaire

(Check off treatments in Appendix C, "Your SHINE Treatment Worksheet.")

### Adrenal Checklist

_____ 1. Hypoglycemia

_____ 2. Shakiness relieved with eating or irritability when hungry

_____ 3. Recurrent sore throats/infections that take a long time to go away

_____ 4. Low blood pressure or frequent dizziness on first standing

_____ 5. Long-term prednisone (cortisone) usage since CFS/FMS began, and feeling better when you took it

If the answer to any of these (1 through 5) is yes, check off #21. Check off #22 if you have day-to-day fatigue. If you have CFS/FMS, also check off #23.

## Thyroid Checklist

_____ 6. Weight gain of more than ten pounds

_____ 7. Low body temperature (under 98 degrees F)

_____ 8. Cold intolerance

_____ 9. Females only: heavy periods

If you are fatigued and the answer to any of these (6 through 9) is yes, check off #19 and ask your physician to consider #20 (unless your free $T_4$ blood test is elevated).

## Iodine Deficiency

_____ 10. Breast cysts or tenderness

If yes and your physician has ruled out breast cancer, check off #18.

## Estrogen (Females Only)

_____ 11. Do you have decreased vaginal lubrication?

_____ 12. Do you have CFS/FMS or severe symptoms of low estrogen that began within three years after you had a hysterectomy, ovaries removed, or a tubal ligation?

_____ 13. Are your symptoms of fatigue, headache, insomnia, or achiness much worse the week before your period?

If the answer to any of these (11 through 13) is yes, check off #24 (unless you have a history of breast cancer or blood clots).

## Vasodepressor Syncope (NMH)—Only in Those with Severe Fatigue and Exercise Intolerance

_____ 14. Do you experience frequent dizziness on standing or low blood pressure (under 100/60)?

_____ 15. Did you ever have a positive tilt-table test?


If the answer to either of these (14 or 15) is yes, discuss with your physician the treatments for NMH and POTS discussed in this chapter.

## Low Testosterone (Males Only)

_____ 16. Do you have CFS/FMS or loss of libido, erectile dysfunction, high blood pressure, high cholesterol, diabetes? If your testosterone blood level is in the lower 30th percentile of the normal range (or higher if the symptoms are especially suggestive), check off #25.

# 6.

# I–Infections: Destroy Your Body's Hidden Invaders

For most people, their key infection is the overgrowth of yeast/candida. I use the terms "yeast," "candida," and "fungal infections" interchangeably.

Because of excess sugar and the increased use of antibiotics, yeast overgrowth is becoming very common in the general population. Add in the immune dysfunction seen in CFS/FMS, and I find that virtually everybody with CFS and fibromyalgia needs to be treated for candida.

Although many lab tests are used for candida, I find most of them to be very unreliable, and I prefer to treat based on symptoms. For most people, this means treating if you have chronic sinusitis or spastic colon. In those with CFS/FMS, I find it is best to simply presume candida overgrowth is present, and treat it.

# Why Is Candida
# Overgrowth So Common?

Most people are familiar with the concept of vaginal yeast overgrowth occurring after antibiotics. It can be hard for people (and physicians) to ignore because there's an obvious discharge. In addition, because there is a test for vaginal yeast overgrowth, physicians are quick to treat it.

Unfortunately, the big problem with candida overgrowth is not in the four inches of vagina, but rather in the twenty-five feet of large and small intestine. Because it does not cause an obvious discharge, and there is no test that distinguishes normal growth from overgrowth, most physicians make believe that bowel candida overgrowth doesn't exist. This is common in medicine, where it seems that "if there is no test for a medical condition, the problem doesn't exist." It reminds me of small children covering their eyes and thinking that they're invisible!

Unfortunately, antibiotics kill off the healthy bacteria that normally live in the colon and allow overgrowth of candida. The body is often able to rebalance itself after one or several courses of antibiotics, but after repeated or long-term courses—and especially if the body has an underlying immune dysfunction—the yeast can get the upper hand. The second major factor? The 140 pounds of sugar per person added to our diet in food processing each year. Yeast grows by fermenting sugar, and if you pour a sixteen-ounce soda, which contains a massive twelve spoonfuls of sugar, down your throat, you're turning your gut into a fermentation tank and creating trillions of little baby yeasties. This contributes to the spastic colon (also called irritable bowel syndrome), which is a hallmark of candida overgrowth. Candida overgrowth is also a major cause of chronic sinusitis. We will discuss both of these below. Let's start by looking at why candida overgrowth can cause widespread immune problems.

## Candida and Immune Function

Fungal overgrowth may suppress the body's immune system. It is suspected that this occurs in part because the bowel yeast infection causes what is called leaky gut syndrome or, to use a more research-based jargon, "increased bowel membrane permeability." Why? Because during part of the candida's life cycle, it grows in threads that can spread into the bowel wall, making it "leaky." This contributes to food proteins getting absorbed into the blood system before they are fully digested. These partially digested proteins will be treated as outside invaders by your immune system. This results in:

1. A marked increase in food allergies and
2. Immune system overactivity (as occurs in autoimmune diseases), combined with immune fatigue.

In addition, as the yeast organism is massive in size compared to viruses or bacteria, it is a difficult bug for your immune system to kill without help once it overgrows. Because of this, once the yeast gets the upper hand, it can up a cycle that further disrupts the body's defenses. Fortunately, once again knowledge is power! So let's look at the information you need to help balance and optimize your immune function.

Yeast is a normal member of the body's "zoo." It lives in balance with bowel bacteria; some bowel bacteria are helpful and healthy, and others are detrimental and unhealthy. The problems begin when this harmonious balance shifts and the yeast begins to overgrow.

# Problems Caused by Candida

Candida can cause a vast variety of symptoms, many of which can be caused by a host of other problems. There are several, however, that leave me presuming candida overgrowth until proven otherwise. These are:

1. Chronic nasal congestion or sinusitis
2. Spastic colon, which is also known as irritable bowel syndrome. This basically means that you have gas, bloating, diarrhea, and/ or constipation and your physician doesn't know why. Although there are several causes, most often when we treat for the candida, the spastic colon goes away!

### • • •   GETTING RID OF CHRONIC SINUSITIS   • • •

Research done at the Mayo Clinic showed that over 90 percent of chronic sinusitis is caused by immune reactivity to fungal growth in the sinuses. The result is a stuffy nose, eventually leading to nasal passages swelling shut. In the body, any time something gets blocked (e.g., an appendix or gallbladder), it results in a secondary bacterial infection—and the sinuses are no exception. When this happens, your nasal mucus turns yellow-green and you go to the doctor in pain. They give you an antibiotic, which knocks out the bacterial infection and leaves you feeling better. Unfortunately, the antibiotic worsens the underlying yeast/fungal infection in your nose, causing more swelling and blockages and therefore more attacks of bacterial infections. Treating sinusitis with antibiotics is why sinusitis in the United States usually becomes chronic.

In my experience, sinusitis (even chronic) usually responds dramatically to the yeast treatments discussed below, especially a combination of six weeks of Diflucan and a special sinusitis nose spray. The spray contains Bactroban and xylitol, which kill the bacterial infections, low-dose cortisol to shrink the swelling, and an antifungal. This combination will often knock out the sinusitis, and some patients like to stay on the nose spray for the long term or use it intermittently for recurrent infections. Your physician can call in a prescription for the sinusitis nose spray to Cape Apothecary 410-757-3522, and Diflucan is available by prescription at any pharmacy.

For those few patients with persistent chronic sinusitis despite treatment, I recommend the book *Sinus Survival* by Robert S. Ivker, a physician whose heart embodies what it means to be a healer (see Appendix E, "Other Resources").

## Treating Yeast/Candida Overgrowth

A number of effective treatments can be used to eliminate yeast overgrowth. I find that the best approach is to combine dietary changes, natural remedies, and prescription medications.

## DIETARY CHANGES AND NATURAL REMEDIES

The most important part of treating yeast overgrowth is avoiding sugar and other sweets, although I will add the three magic words, "except for chocolate." You can also enjoy one or two pieces of fruit a day, but don't consume concentrated sugars like fruit juices, corn syrup, jellies, pastry, candy, or honey. Stay far away from soft drinks, which have nine teaspoons of sugar in every twelve ounces. This amount of sugar has been shown to markedly suppress immune function for several hours. Be prepared to go through sugar withdrawal for about one week when you cut sugar out of your diet. My book *Beat Sugar Addiction Now* can help you become a recovered sugar addict—easily!

Using stevia as a sweetener is a wonderful substitute for sugar. Despite some misconceptions, stevia is safe and natural, and you can use all you want. The brand of stevia that you choose is important, however. Many brands of stevia are not filtered and therefore are bitter. Several excellent Stevia brands include Body Ecology (1-800-4-stevia), SweetLeaf, and Stevita. In addition, Truvia and Pure Via, which are made by Coke- and Pepsi-affiliated companies, are also good sugar substitutes.

There are now even several good soda substitutes. Hansen's diet sodas (sweetened with Splenda) and Zevia sodas (sweetened with stevia) are reasonable. Interestingly, Coke and Pepsi recently came out with, and I thought I would never say this, healthy lines of soft drinks. Look for their Vitaminwater and SoBe sugar-free, zero-calorie sodas that are sweetened with stevia. When I first saw these, I read through the ingredients, waiting to find the usual "poisons." When I got to the bottom of the list I was shocked not to have found any, and even went back and read the list again. These are actually reasonably healthy soda substitutes. My favorite? Go with the Vitaminwater Zero Go-Go Mixed Berry, which even has some ribose in it!

Several books have been written on the yeast controversy and offer additional dietary methods to try. One of the best is *The Yeast Connection and the Woman* by the late Dr. William Crook, a remarkable physician who introduced and advanced our understanding of candida overgrowth. His work is so important that he is one of the three physicians to whom this book is dedicated!

Many books on yeast overgrowth, including Dr. Crook's book, advise readers to avoid all yeast. This information is based on the theory that an allergic reaction to yeast is the cause of the problem. However, the yeast that is found in most foods (except beer and cheese) is not closely related to candida, which is the predominant yeast that seems to be involved in yeast overgrowth.

In my experience, trying to avoid all yeast in foods results in a nutritionally inadequate diet and does not substantially help most people. Although a few people do appear to have true allergies to the yeast in their food, they account for a small percentage of my patients with suspected yeast overgrowth. These people may benefit from the stricter diet recommended in Dr. Crook's books. Interestingly, once adrenal insufficiency and yeast overgrowth are treated, most people find that their allergies and sensitivities to yeast and other food products seem to improve and often disappear.

## SUPPLEMENTS TO TREAT CANDIDA

1. Healthy gut bacteria compete with candida. This is why probiotics are so helpful. Unfortunately, over 99 percent of these healthy bacteria are usually killed by stomach acid, so they don't put up much of a fight. Because of this, I recommend that the probiotics be taken in an enteric coated form, such as the "pearl" form. These pearls act like tanks that carry the probiotics past the stomach acid safely and then dissolve in the alkaline environment of the intestines, releasing your healthy bacteria "troops" to fight the candida. I recommend a brand called Pearls Elite by Enzymatic Therapy, although a new product called Primadophilus Optima, by Nature's Way, is looking like it may be even better, with 90 billion healthy bacteria in an enteric capsule. Take one of either each day for five months, and then every other day as needed to maintain bowel health.

2. There are many natural products that fight candida. I recommend Lauricidin, discussed below under viral infections (see page 142), which kills off many unwanted bugs, and is a good idea for anyone with candida or CFS/FMS.

## PRESCRIPTION TREATMENTS FOR YEAST OVERGROWTH

1. It is critical to add a prescription antifungal because the natural products only kill yeast in the gut and are often not strong enough on their own. I routinely recommend that those with chronic si-

nusitis, spastic colon, or CFS/FMS take the medication Diflucan (fluconazole) at a dose of 200 milligrams a day for six to twelve weeks. You will need a holistic physician to prescribe this.

If symptoms of yeast overgrowth are caused by an allergic or sensitivity reaction to the yeast body parts, symptoms may flare up when mass quantities of the yeast are suddenly killed off. This is called a die-off (Herxheimer) reaction and can occur with the treatment of any chronic infection. To decrease the risk of this reaction, start your treatment with the probiotics and Lauricidin (using the dosing regimen on page 142) for three to four weeks before starting the Diflucan. If symptoms flare on the Diflucan, I stop the medication until the reaction subsides and then lower the dose to 25 to 100 milligrams each morning for the first three to fourteen days. If symptoms recur after stopping the Diflucan, I may continue the medication for an additional six weeks at 200 milligrams a day, or even, in severe cases, prescribe 200 milligrams twice a day one day a week over the long term to keep the candida suppressed. This is especially helpful if the person is on long treatment with antibiotics. Those with a severe Herxheimer reaction may want to consider also trying a yeast-free diet for six to twelve weeks to see if this helps.

2. For people with chronic nasal congestion or sinusitis, I add a prescription sinusitis nose spray from Cape Apothecary (410-757-3522). I have them take one spray in each nostril twice a day for one bottle and then as needed. Patients love it!

The best thing you can do to combat yeast overgrowth is to try to avoid it in the first place. When you get an infection, immediately begin treating it naturally (see "Treating Infections Without Antibiotics" below). Hopefully, you will be able to prevent it from turning into a bacterial infection that might require an antibiotic.

If you find, however, that you must take an antibiotic, all is not lost. You can still lessen the severity of yeast overgrowth by avoiding sweets and by taking Lauricidin plus a probiotic.

## TREATING INFECTIONS WITHOUT ANTIBIOTICS

Many people do not realize how many things they can do before resorting to using an antibiotic to clear an infection. If you feel you are coming down with a respiratory infection such as a cold or the flu, I recommend that you try the following:

- *Take natural thymic hormone.* This is available as a product called ProBoost (see pages 141 and 287), and it is an outstanding immune stimulant. Dissolve the contents of one packet under your tongue three times a day and let it get absorbed there (any that is swallowed will be destroyed by your stomach acid). I recommend that this be in everyone's medicine cabinet and should be begun immediately at the start of any infection.
- *Take 1,000 milligrams of vitamin C a day.*
- *Suck on a 20-milligram zinc acetate lozenge (or other zinc if acetate not available) four times a day.*
- *Drink plenty of water and hot caffeine-free tea (or hot water with lemon) and rest!*

- *If you have a sinus infection, try nasal rinses.* Dissolve one-half teaspoon of salt in a cup of lukewarm water. Add a pinch of baking soda to make it more soothing. Inhale some of the solution about one inch up into your nose, one nostril at a time. Do this either by using a baby nose bulb or an eyedropper while lying down, or by sniffing the solution out of the palm of your hand while standing by a sink. Then gently blow your nose, being careful not to hurt your ears. Repeat the same process with the other nostril. Continue to repeat with each nostril until the nose is clear. Rinse your nasal passages at least twice a day until the infection improves. Each rinsing will wash away about 90 percent of the infection and make it much easier for your body to heal.
- *Gargle* with salt water, mixed as described above for the nasal rinse, to help a sore throat.
- Bladder infections can often be prevented or eliminated with the supplement mannose.

## WHAT IF THE YEAST COMES BACK?

The best marker that I have found for recurrent yeast overgrowth is a return of bowel symptoms, with gas, bloating, and/or diarrhea or constipation; vaginal yeast; mouth sores; and/or recurring nasal congestion or sinusitis. If these symptoms persist for more than two to three weeks, consider repeating the yeast treatment.

# Why Are We Seeing Increasing Immune Problems?

In addition to new infections arriving on the scene (e.g., AIDS, swine flu, Lyme disease, and a host of others), we are also seeing a rising epidemic of autoimmune diseases. Autoimmune illness occurs when part of the person's own body is mistaken for an outside invader, and it is attacked by the immune system. There are literally hundreds of autoimmune conditions, including multiple sclerosis, lupus, rheumatoid arthritis, and Hashimoto's thyroiditis—and they are becoming markedly more common.

## • • • IS IT LUPUS, OR REALLY FIBROMYALGIA? • • •

Lupus is an autoimmune illness where the body's immune system confuses it with an outside invader and attacks itself. It can be mild, or severe and life threatening.

A key problem is that lupus, and many other autoimmune illnesses like rheumatoid arthritis and Sjögren's syndrome, frequently cause a secondary fibromyalgia, which is often missed. Many if not most of the symptoms may then be caused by the secondary fibromyalgia and do not respond to the standard autoimmune medications, so the doctor gives higher and higher doses of prednisone and other toxic treatments.

So how can you tell? If you have widespread pain and fatigue, and also insomnia, you likely have a secondary fibromyalgia that should also be treated with SHINE.

In addition, for those with lupus, several studies have shown that 200 milligrams a day (a large dose for women) of DHEA improves outcomes in lupus. Though this high dose would sometimes cause acne or darkening of facial hair in women, in the studies this was uncommon in those with lupus.

## Why the Autoimmune Epidemic?

It is important to step back and once again look at some of the root causes.

Why are so many people's immune systems becoming overwhelmed?

In addition to sleep deprivation and nutritional deficiencies (especially zinc and vitamin D) contributing to immune dysfunction, there are several other major underlying factors that are becoming very common in the population as a whole:

1. *Severe dysbiosis (unhealthy gut infections) caused by antibiotics, excess sugar intake, and acid blockers.* With a normal bowel containing more organisms than the entire rest of our body, the widespread growth of toxic organisms in the colon is a major problem. To put this in perspective, it used to be that when babies were born they were breast-fed, developed a colon full of healthy bacteria, and then developed stomach acid that kept out all other bacteria. There were no antibiotics, acid blockers, or massive amounts of sugar added to the diet to later disrupt this healthy ecosystem, so it stayed in a healthy balance for the rest of people's lives.

2. *Incomplete digestion of proteins caused by the rapidly increasing and chronic use of acid-blocker medication, combined with the routine destruction of the enzymes present in food during food processing to prolong shelf life.* These enzymes are what digest food completely, and deficiencies result in incompletely digested proteins.

3. *Increased gut membrane permeability,* often called leaky gut, allowing dramatic increases in absorption of these partially digested proteins, which, as discussed above, are treated by your immune system as outside invaders.

This trio of modern-day gut changes not only contributes to a marked increase in food allergies, and likely autoimmune disease, but can also overwhelm and exhaust the immune system. Why? If you consider that the total body burden of many infections may be measured in under a milligram, and that people may eat upward of 100,000 milligrams of protein a day, the concern is raised that even modest decreases in protein digestion, and the absorption of a small percent of partially digested amino acid chains, may increase the immune system's work dramatically.

### • • •   OUR MODERN DIGESTIVE DISASTER   • • •

Unfortunately, food processors learned that by destroying the digestive enzymes in food, they could prolong the food's shelf life. This is because the enzymes in the food cause the food to ripen. The same enzymes, however, are necessary for you to properly digest your food. So the food looks good on the shelf, but it is difficult to digest, causing indigestion. Instead of treating the poor digestion by giving people digestive enzymes, physicians instead turn off stomach acid—the other major factor needed for digestion. This is like going to your physician saying that you have a flat tire, and having them shoot out the other tire to restore balance. Not a good idea. So if you have indigestion, take some plant-based digestive enzymes with your meals (e.g., CompleteGest by Enzymatic Therapy) and improve stomach acidity. This will be discussed in chapter 7, "N—Nutrition: Optimizing Your Body's Ability to Heal, Including Ribose, a Powerful New Nutrient." To again put this in perspective and help you understand the stress that poor digestion puts on your immune system, consider this thought. It would take over 20,000 trillion viruses to equal the weight of the amount of protein in a hamburger. So you want to improve your digestion so that your stomach digests the burger. Otherwise, the partially digested proteins will have to be eliminated by your immune system, sometimes exhausting and overwhelming it.

To give an idea of the impact of these food sensitivities, a recently published study funded by our foundation showed that twenty-three of thirty autistic children were able to return to regular schools after one year of food allergy desensitization treatments with NAET (Nambudripad's Allergy Elimination Technique) versus zero out of thirty in the untreated control group. Interestingly, many researchers in the field are seeing overlaps in the pathophysiology of autism and fibromyalgia.

## ANOTHER MAJOR CAUSE OF AUTOIMMUNE DISEASE

We now have over 85,000 chemicals added to our environment that were not there one hundred years ago. To get a chemical approved as a medication, it has to go through the safety evaluation process that costs many millions of dollars. On the other hand, if you just want to throw the chemical wildly into the environment, it is okay to do so without any real safety testing. An example gaining more attention is Bisphenol A (BPA), a chemical found in plastic and metal food containers. Over one hundred studies are showing that it can be very toxic and, like DDT (dichlorodiphenyltrichloroethane), acts as a hormone disrupter. Those of you old enough to remember DDT may also remember that it nearly drove our national symbol, the bald eagle, to extinction before it was outlawed. Though BPA has been banned in Canada, it is still allowed to be used in the United States.

It is likely that this chemical load is one more major contributing factor that can result in the immune system confusing its own body's parts with outside invaders. It is neither possible nor recommended that all chemicals be avoided. Rather, simply trim back your overall exposure using common sense. For those with severe autoimmune illness, I recommend an excellent book called *The Autoimmune Epidemic* by Donna Jackson Nakazawa.

# Supporting Your Immune System

Fortunately, our bodies (including our immune systems) are built with a remarkable ability to adapt, especially if they are given a bit of help. Let's start with a few key things that are critical in helping your immune function.

## NUTRITION

As we will discuss in chapter 7, widespread nutritional deficiencies are very common in modern life. Many of these can contribute to immune dysfunction. Especially important? A simple mineral called zinc. Along with vitamin D, this mineral is one of the most important nutrients for optimal immune function. Unfortunately, with chronic infections or inflammation zinc gets used up and lost in the urine, resulting in zinc deficiency. This is commonly seen in AIDS patients, where the zinc deficiency is so severe that it can account for many, if not most, of the immune dysfunction seen early in the illness. Research has shown that fibromyalgia patients also are zinc deficient, which is no surprise given their chronic infections.

Fortunately, zinc is cheap, costing a few pennies a day. Unfortunately, because it is cheap, you are not going to hear much advertising about how important it is. Treatment is simple. In most people, the Energy Revitalization System vitamin powder (see chapter 7) will be enough to maintain healthy zinc levels. So that's an easy one. Other nutrients are also very important for immune function, including vitamins A, C, D, and other nutrients. These are all present in the vitamin powder, or many good multivitamins, keeping this easy.

In addition to taking a good multivitamin with zinc, other key points for optimizing your immune function include:

1. Cut back excess sugar. The amount of sugar in a twelve-ounce can of soda will suppress immune function by 30 percent for three hours.
2. Get adequate sleep.
3. Optimize adrenal function.
4. Improve digestion with a plant-based digestive enzyme.

All of these take a major load off your immune system, so it can get back to its real job of getting rid of the bad guys.

## INFECTIONS—INTENSIVE CARE FOR THOSE WITH CFS/FMS

For those of you with CFS/FMS, welcome to the "Infection of the Month Club."

Many of you have noticed that there seems to be a regular flow of new infections that get blamed for CFS and fibromyalgia. I have watched this occur over and over in the last thirty years, with literally dozens of different infections being blamed as "the cause." So CFS/FMS is generally not occurring from a single infection—but rather most people have many infections that are dragging them down.

Immune dysfunction is an integral part of chronic fatigue syndrome and fibromyalgia. In fact, some people use the name CFIDS, or chronic fatigue and *immune dysfunction* syndrome, instead of CFS.

Because of the immune dysfunction, people with CFS pick up many "hitchhiker" infections. In addition, there are many viral infections, such as infectious mononucleosis (EBV or Epstein-Barr Virus), HHV-6 (human herpesvirus 6), CMV (cytomegalovirus), herpes zoster (aka chickenpox and shingles), and others that are never entirely cleared from our body once we have them—and most people have had these infections by the time they're twenty years old. For these infections, and others, the body often finds it easier to simply lock up the last remaining viruses in little jail cells where they stay for the rest of our lives.

Unless our immune function goes down, in which case there is sometimes a jailbreak. Then we have what is called "viral reactivation."

Unfortunately, although testing is very good at picking up most acute first-time infections, it is very unreliable at diagnosing chronic infections. So deciding whether to treat for infections in CFS/FMS is best based on symptoms and response to treatment rather than simply relying on the testing.

The good news? It is not necessary to track down and kill every infection. Almost all of these infections are what are considered "opportunistic" infections. By definition, this means that they cannot survive when your immune system is healthy. Because of this, once you have cleared out a few key infections and help your immune system to heal, it knows how to get rid of the rest of the infections.

There are certain infections in which the organisms are, simply put, massive in size. For example, by way of comparison, if a virus was the size of the period at a end of this sentence, a candida (fungal) thread could be the size of a house. And some parasites would be even larger. We will teach you how to knock out these big bad bugs, so your immune system can take care of the little guys.

There are literally dozens of infections implicated in CFS/FMS, and the most important ones to deal with fall under four categories:

1. Candida/yeast infections (discussed above)
2. Parasites
3. Antibiotic-sensitive infections
4. Viral infections

In addition, in some cases, it is not the infection itself but your body's reaction to it that causes your symptoms. As we noted above, a desensitization technique called NAET was very effective for helping in autism by treating allergies and sensitivities in our recently published study. NAET has also been very helpful for treating allergies and sensitivities in people with CFS/FMS, sometimes even making their illness go away. We are hopeful that this desensitization technique may also help with the infections seen in CFS/FMS. More on NAET in chapter 10 under "Check for Food Allergies."

## Step 1—Kill Off Candida

How to do this was discussed earlier in this chapter.

## Step 2—Kill Off Bowel Parasites

Although we often think of parasites as just a problem encountered when traveling, infection by giardia, amoebae, and numerous other bowel parasites is common in the United States. In fact, in my initial study, one out of six people with CFS/FMS had a parasite, and parasites have been shown to be one of the many causes of CFS/FMS.

## DIAGNOSING BOWEL PARASITES

Most standard laboratories are clueless about how to do proper stool testing for parasites and will miss the vast majority of these infections. Testing has to be done at a lab that specializes in parasitology. These include the following labs:

1. Parasitology Center Inc. Parasite testing is what they do. Especially for those on a limited budget, this is where I would send the stool specimen (www.parasitetesting.com). I would order the Comprehensive Stool Analysis Test (CPT 87177). This offers the information I find most helpful.
2. Genova Diagnostics. This lab has a wide array of holistic tests (www.gdx.net).
3. Diagnos-Techs, Doctor's Data, and several other specialty labs can also be helpful.

When getting the stool sample, it has to be a loose, watery stool (i.e., one that takes the shape of the specimen container). Taking one or two Dulcolax tablets the night before is helpful if you don't routinely have loose stools. At the same time, collect a second stool specimen to test for a special bowel infection called *Clostridium difficile*, which makes a toxin that can also trigger CFS/FMS. The stool test for *Clostridium difficile* toxin, fortunately, can be done well at any lab, making it more likely to be covered by insurance. The sample for *Clostridium difficile* (which is often simply called *C. diff.*) needs to be taken to the lab within two hours or frozen. The other samples for the parasites are sent to one of the labs above and the directions will be included in the specimen kit that you order from the lab (with your health practitioner's prescription) before collecting the specimen.

## TREATING BOWEL PARASITES

Common parasites include giardia, blastocystis, and amebic infections. The appropriate treatment for bowel parasites depends on which organism is causing the problem. Some doctors will consider some parasites to be "nonpathogenic." This means they don't necessarily cause bowel problems unless a person has immune dysfunction. Because people with CFS/FMS have immune dysfunction, I find it important to treat all parasite infections—and people usually feel considerably better when the parasite is eliminated. In addition, when a parasitic infection is suspected, but no parasites can be found in the lab testing, I sometimes consider treating the person empirically with Alinia (nitazoxanide), 1,000 milligrams twice a day for ten days. This covers a large number of bowel infections. Warning—this is quite expensive, so check to be sure it is covered by your prescription insurance plan.

### THE IMPORTANCE OF FILTERING WATER

Water filters can be helpful in the fight against parasitic infection and can help to improve health in general. However, not all units are designed to filter out parasites. In fact, it seems that many, if not most, water filters seem to do very little. For those interested in a high-quality yet reasonably priced water filter,

I recommend Bren Jacobson, my favorite water expert (www .jacobsonhealth.com or 410-224-4877). For drinking water, the Multipure filters are most cost effective. Reverse osmosis plus carbon block whole-house filters can also be very effective but are expensive.

# Step 3—Kill Off Viral Infections

There are many viruses that have been implicated in CFS/FMS. The most important are:

1. HHV-6 (human herpesvirus 6)
2. EBV (Epstein-Barr virus)
3. CMV (cytomegalovirus)

It is possible that viruses that affect the gastrointestinal tract may join this list in the future.

## TESTING

The standard tests for these viruses include an IgM antibody, which usually only goes up in the first two to three months after the *initial* infection. Because in CFS/FMS these represent viral reactivation, and generally not the initial infection, this test is fairly useless in CFS/FMS. Meanwhile, the IgG antibody tests for these viruses will be positive in over 90 percent of healthy adults, as this test simply shows that you had this infection in the past. So a positive IgG antibody test by itself is also relatively meaningless. On the other hand, research is suggesting that very high levels of the IgG antibody may suggest viral reactivation. Because of this, if the IgG antibody for the HHV-6 or CMV virus is greater than 4 (or 1:640 or greater, which is another way these tests may be reported), I am more likely to suspect a reactivated viral infection that needs treatment, especially if the person is not feeling adequately improved with other treatments by four to six months. I no longer find the EBV (Epstein-Barr virus) tests to be helpful. Instead, I use the symptoms below to decide whether to use an antiviral despite the HHV-6 or CMV tests being normal.

## SYMPTOMS

I am more likely to suspect an important underlying viral infection if:

1. The person's CFS/FMS began with a severe flu-like illness and persists despite SHINE.
2. The person has pure CFS with predominantly flu-like symptoms, with debilitating fatigue and little or no pain, or with low blood pressure symptoms (NMH/POTS—see chapter 5).

## ANTIVIRAL TREATMENTS

Antivirals are only needed in about 5 to 10 percent of CFS patients. The main antiviral I am using is Valcyte (valganciclovir), giving 900 milligrams twice a day for three weeks, followed by 900 milligrams once a day for twenty-three weeks. It is effective against CMV, HHV-6, and EBV viruses. It can take four months to see the benefits, and some people will initially have a *die-off reaction* where their CFS/FMS symptoms worsen for the first few weeks to months of treatment as dead virus parts are released into their system. This medication is extremely expensive (approximately $24,000 a year), so I generally will not use it unless there's prescription coverage.

Another antiviral that is much less expensive and can also be helpful is Imunovir (inosine pranobex). It is very reasonable to use this before the Valcyte if one cannot get it covered by insurance.

## IMUNOVIR/ISOPRINOSINE FOR VIRAL INFECTIONS

### Recommended Dosage

The prescribed dosage is one 500-milligram capsule twice a day Monday through Friday with none on the weekend. The following week the dose is three capsules twice a day Monday through Friday with none on the weekend. Then, none the following week. Then repeat the cycle—staying on for two three-week cycles and off one.

### Precautions

Very safe and approved in many countries except the United States (but it can still be shipped to the United States). There can be a temporary rise in uric acid (so be careful if you have gout). However, uric acid is low in most CFS patients and acts as an antioxidant, so this may actually be beneficial.

*(continued)*

**Source**

Can be obtained on an individual basis for patients from Canada. Fax the prescription and order form filled out by your physician to Rivex Pharma at (800) 784-0976.

Prescription should read:

Isoprinosine/Imunovir 500 milligrams
Sig: as directed
# bottles, and refills
ICD-9 780.71 Dx: CFS
On special request for personal import only

Note: The cost is $205 for a bottle of one hundred plus $20 for shipping. With above dosing, patients will use one and one-third bottle (130 caps) every three months.

Another treatment that may be helpful for chronic viral infections is vitamin C. High doses of 15 to 50 grams of vitamin C, administered intravenously, are often dramatically helpful for CFS when given as part of intravenous nutritional therapy that your holistic doctor may administer. They may also add the antiviral glycyrrhizin, which is the active agent in licorice.

Last but not least, studies are suggesting that antibody deficiencies (called IgG subtypes) are very common in CFS/FMS and may contribute to both the immune dysfunction and nerve pain. Giving gamma globulin (antibodies from human blood donors) intramuscularly (2 cc IM weekly or 4 cc IM every other week for six weeks) has been very helpful for CFS/FMS patients. It also costs much less than giving it intravenously or subcutaneously. Unfortunately, there are periods where the intramuscular gamma globulin is hard to obtain, as it gets used up by the military to fight and prevent wartime infections. In those cases, and especially if insurance coverage is available (cost can be upward of $30,000 a year, versus about $600 for the gamma globulin IM series), the subcutaneous or intravenous gamma globulin injections may be very helpful. The infusions have the added benefit of helping severe nerve pain (see pages 196 and 211). The use of gamma globulin in CFS/FMS is being researched by a number of scientists, including Mark Sivieri, M.D., an excellent CFS/FMS specialist in Laurel, Maryland.

## • • • TWO POWERFUL NATURAL ANTIVIRALS • • •

In addition to these prescription antivirals, there are also several other natural treatments that may be helpful in fighting viral infections in CFS.

1. Thymic protein A, marketed under the brand name Pro-Boost, is an excellent natural immune stimulant. Although not a hormone, thymic protein A mimics the natural hormone produced by the thymus, the gland that stimulates the immune system. I find it to be extraordinarily effective in fighting common acute infections of any kind that seem to pop up, and I recommend that it be in everyone's medicine cabinet. In fact, whenever my kids would get a cold, the first thing they'd say is, "Dad, where's the white powder [the Pro-Boost]?"

*(continued)*

Although taking it for one to three days will quickly eliminate most acute viral infections, for the chronic viral infections seen in CFS, one packet three times a day for three months is needed. In one study, this dropped EBV IgG levels by 70 percent after three months in CFS patients.

2. Monolaurin. Lauric acid, from coconut oil, was first discovered as an antiviral and antibacterial substance in human breast milk. It is more effective (and less likely to cause acid reflux) when combined with glycerol, forming monolaurin. Monolaurin has been shown to be active against a number of viruses and bacteria, and likely also has antifungal activity, making it very promising in CFS/FMS. I routinely use it as a first-line treatment in anyone with candida or other chronic infections. It is nonprescription and very reasonably priced. It comes as Lauricidin, which is monolaurin in an easy-to-use and lower-cost micropellet form.

## How to Take Lauricidin

Take Lauricidin with or after meals. The micropellets can be placed in the mouth and swallowed with water. Do not chew or take with hot liquids, as it will taste oily. It can be potent enough against the infections to trigger a die-off reaction at high doses, so you may want to begin slowly, at 750 milligrams (one-quarter blue scoop) or less, one to two times daily for a week before increasing the amount. The level can then be increased to 1.5 grams (one half blue scoop), one to two times a day. One container is enough to tell if it will help.

Both of these are available without prescription at www.end fatigue.com.

As you can see, there are a number of antiviral treatments. Higher cost does not necessarily mean more effective results, and it is best to tailor therapy to each individual case.

## Antibiotic-Sensitive Infections

These are infections that improve when the person gets an antibiotic, suggesting a hidden infection. If any of these five are present, I recommend antibiotic treatment:

1. A fever over 98.6°F—even 99°F, as most people with CFS/FMS have a low temperature;

2. Chronic lung congestion;

3. A history of bad reactions to several different antibiotics (people misinterpret this die-off reaction as an allergic reaction—but being "allergic" to several unrelated antibiotics but not to other medications is quite unlikely);

4. Scabbing scalp sores—for these cases, the antibiotic Zithromax (azithromycin) has been found to be helpful;

5. A history of vertigo lasting over three months (in which case I suspect Lyme disease, which can irritate the nerve serving the middle ear balance centers). Dizziness and disequilibrium without a feeling of spinning in a circle is common in CFS/FMS and does not count as vertigo.

Unfortunately, there are no reliable tests for most of these antibiotic-sensitive infections, whether they be mycoplasma, Lyme disease, or a host of others. Most testing is either hopelessly unlikely to find the infection when present, or is likely to find the infection in everybody. I do not consider any of them to be especially useful at this time, although the standard Lyme Western Blot test and antibody screening tests done at most standard labs should be treated if positive in people with CFS/FMS.

Lyme disease is especially problematic, as there is *no* gold standard test. I suspect that over half of the people who have Lyme infections have negative tests and, conversely, if you randomly check Lyme tests, as many as half of the people who test positive do not have Lyme disease. This creates enormous confusion, as CFS/FMS symptoms are similar to those of Lyme disease. Because of this, many people desperately looking for an explanation for their symptoms who have found one of many Lyme tests to be positive cling to this diagnosis as they seek an explanation for their disability. Many of these patients feel better on antibiotics and take this as confirmation. Indeed, many excellent physicians who specialize in treating CFS/FMS feel that the large majority of CFS/FMS patients have Lyme disease. Unfortunately, the majority of CFS/FMS-illiterate physicians only believe a Lyme infection is present if a test called the Western Blot is positive—ignoring that this test has clearly been shown to be negative in a very large percentage of those with Lyme disease.

Given all of the above, we simply do not know for sure how many people with CFS/FMS also have Lyme disease. If you have a history of tick bite associated with a "bull's-eye" rash and have fatigue or pain, I consider it reasonable to treat for possible Lyme disease, even if the tests are negative. The approach I currently recommend (until we have better testing) is to simply acknowledge that the testing used in CFS/FMS patients for antibiotic-sensitive infections in general is unreliable, that the research shows that these infections are common in CFS/FMS, and that the research also shows that many patients improve when given antibiotics such as azithromycin (Zithromax) or doxycycline—even if testing is negative. Given this situation, it is reasonable for physicians to use their clinical judgment and treat with antibiotics when appropriate, even if there is no test to confirm the type of infection.

# Treating the Hidden
# Antibiotic-Sensitive Infections

People with the symptoms discussed above seem to be more likely to have infections that respond to special antibiotics. The antibiotics most likely to affect these organisms are the following:

*Doxycycline or, preferably, minocycline, usually at dosages of 100 milligrams twice a day.* These two antibiotics are in the tetracycline family. These antibiotics should not be given to children under eight years of age because they can cause permanent staining of the teeth.

*Ciprofloxacin (Cipro), usually 500 to 750 milligrams twice a day.* This antibiotic has a wide range of effectiveness against a large number of organisms. Cipro has an additional benefit for men, as it also treats any hidden prostate infections, as does doxycycline. You should not take oral magnesium or any supplement containing magnesium within four to six hours of taking Cipro or you may not absorb the Cipro as completely. A small percentage of the population has a genetic defect that prevents them from breaking down Cipro. In this group, taking Cipro can actually trigger FMS, and this family of antibiotics should be avoided if you are related to someone who developed fibromyalgia after taking Cipro.

*Azithromycin (Zithromax), 250 to 500 milligrams a day.* These antibiotics are in the erythromycin family. Zithromax tends to be fairly well tolerated. Begin with this antibiotic if you have scalp or skin sores or scabs.

If you do have low-grade chronic temperature elevations, be sure that you monitor your temperature during treatment. If your temperature drops with the antibiotic, it suggests that you do have one of these antibiotic-sensitive infections and that the antibiotic is helping. This would encourage me to continue the antibiotic trial—even if it takes up to eighteen months to see an improvement in your symptoms.

If you are clearly better, you should probably take the antibiotic for at least six to twelve months. It can then be stopped. If symptoms recur, keep repeating six- to eight-week cycles until the symptoms stay gone. It may take several years of treatment for the infection to be totally eradicated. To put this in perspective, this is how long children often take antibiotics for acne—which, unfortunately, if not taken with antifungals, can lead to yeast overgrowth and possibly trigger CFS/FMS. You should therefore take a good probiotic such as Pearls Elite once a day. I'll sometimes add Diflucan, 200 milligrams twice a day, one day a week, as well. Also, be aware that birth control pills may be ineffective while you are taking antibiotics, so be sure to use an alternative form of birth control.

Occasionally, people get what is called a die-off (Herxheimer) reaction as the infection dies off. This occurs when the proteins are released from destroyed infection more quickly than the body can eliminate them. Killing infections can also trigger release of immune system chemicals called cytokines. These can flare symptoms that include chills, fever, night sweats, and muscle pain, along with generally worsening CFS/FMS symptoms as the antibiotic first kills off the infection. Many people mistakenly confuse these with an allergic reaction. These symptoms can be severe and can last for weeks. I stop the antibiotic, let the die-off reaction subside, and then resume the antibiotic at a much lower dose (e.g., 25 milligrams of minocycline every other day) and work the dose up slowly. Taking anti-inflammatory herbs such as willow bark, boswellia, and curcumin (End Pain and/or Curamin) may also help. Dr. Garth Nicolson, who pioneered this treatment of antibiotic-sensitive infections in CFS/FMS, notes that if you have been sick for years, it is unlikely that you will recover in less than one year of treatment, so you should not be alarmed by symptoms that return or worsen temporarily. In addition, some other unusual infections may require the simultaneous use of multiple antibiotics. Fortunately, using the entire SHINE protocol along with the antibiotics often results in improvement being seen within three to four months of antibiotic use, and persisting when the antibiotics are stopped. This makes SHINE especially important in those with chronic Lyme infections.

## Bowel Bacterial Infections

One more antibiotic-sensitive infection deserves special mention. If spastic colon symptoms persist after treatment for yeast and parasites, consider treating for SIBO (small intestinal bacterial overgrowth), which is common in CFS/FMS and which is another key cause of bowel symptoms attributed to irritable bowel syndrome. SIBO occurs when bacteria migrate upstream from the colon (large intestine), where they belong, to the small intestine. Normally, the bowel contractions that move food downstream also wash bacteria out of the small intestine. If these normal contractions are weakened, as occurs with an underactive thyroid, SIBO is more likely. Often, simply optimizing thyroid hormone levels can help. If needed, research has shown that treating spastic colon/SIBO empirically with the antibiotic rifaximin (Xifaxan), 400 to 550 milligrams three times a day for ten days, can result in long-lasting improvement. This antibiotic is quite expensive, so if not covered by insurance I will sometimes substitute neomycin, 500-milligram tablets three times a day for ten days.

In summary, many infections can cause or be caused by CFS and FMS. These are usually associated with immune system malfunction. Testing for most infections is both expensive and not reliable, though there are a few that I consider worthwhile. These include stool testing for parasites (done only at a few labs specializing in parasitology) and blood testing for HHV-6 and CMV viral infections, checking only the IgG antibody levels (see recommended lab tests in chapter 13). Beyond these, it is reasonable to treat empirically based on symptoms— that is, without testing. If you have lung congestion and/or recurrent temperatures over 98.6°F, scalp scabs, vertigo, or a history of repeated "allergic" reactions to multiple antibiotics, or if your CFS/FMS improved with antibiotics in the past, your doctor may be able to effectively treat you with antibiotics. If you have chronic flu-like symptoms or if your illness began with a flu-like infection, and your blood tests show very elevated CMV or HHV–6 IgG antibodies (at 1:640 or higher, or over 4), I consider antiviral treatment with Imunovir or Valcyte, but usually only if symptoms persist after treating with the rest of SHINE. Fortunately, there are now physicians around the country who can expertly guide you through these therapies (see chapter 13, "Finding a Physician, Lab Tests, and Other Helpful Tools"). More detailed information on infections in CFS/FMS can be found in *From Fatigued to Fantastic!* Our new understanding of how to diagnose and treat the infections offers exciting new hope.

## Should I Get the Flu Vaccine?

I think it is a good idea for those over sixty-five or folks with a serious medical condition to get the regular flu vaccine each year and the pneumonia vaccine every five years as well after age sixty-five. I currently consider the swine flu vaccines to be a bad idea, unless conditions change markedly.

The regular flu vaccine is a double-edged sword for people with CFS/FMS. In some patients, it can cause mild flu-like symptoms for a few days or, in rare cases, a severe flare-up of symptoms. Still, unless you are one of the 10 percent of CFS/FMS patients who feel worse after the flu shot or other vaccinations, it is reasonable to get a flu shot each year. Otherwise, for most people, it is a matter of personal preference. Basically, take it if you feel like it.

## Important Points

1. Immune problems are escalating because of many problems.
2. For most people, the key infection to treat would be

candida/yeast overgrowth if you have chronic sinusitis or spastic colon.

3. Overall, a good multivitamin and optimizing sleep and digestion are keys to improving immunity.

4. In CFS/FMS, specific sets of symptoms may point to the need to use antibiotics or antivirals.

## Questionnaire

(Check off treatments in Appendix C, "Your SHINE Treatment Worksheet.")

### Yeast/Candida Infections

_____ 1. Do you have sinusitis, nasal congestion, or spastic colon?
  If yes to any of these, check off #26, 27, and 28. If yes to sinusitis, check off #34 and skip question #2.

_____ 2. Yeast Questionnaire

The total score for this section gives the probability of yeast overgrowth being a significant factor in your case.

### Point Score (Add Up and Put Total Below)

50 _____ Have you been treated for acne with tetracycline, erythromycin, or any other antibiotic for one month or longer?

50 _____ Have you taken antibiotics for any type of infection for more than two consecutive months, or shorter courses more than three times in a twelve-month period?

5 _____ Have you ever taken an antibiotic—even for a single course?

25 \_\_\_\_ Have you ever had prostatitis or vaginitis?

5 \_\_\_\_ Have you ever been pregnant?

15 \_\_\_\_ Have you taken birth control pills?

15 \_\_\_\_ Have you taken corticosteroids such as prednisone, Cortef, or Medrol?

15 \_\_\_\_ When you are exposed to perfumes, insecticides, or other odors or chemicals, do you develop wheezing, burning eyes, or any other distress?

20 \_\_\_\_ Are your symptoms worse on damp or humid days or in moldy places?

20 \_\_\_\_ Have you ever had a fungal infection such as jock itch, athlete's foot, or a nail or skin infection that was difficult to treat?

20 \_\_\_\_ Do you crave sugar or breads?

10 \_\_\_\_ Does tobacco smoke cause you discomfort (e.g., wheezing, burning eyes)?

Total:

If 70 or higher, check off #26, 27, and 28.

## For Those with CFS/FMS ONLY

### PARASITES

\_\_\_\_ 3. Did your problems begin with a diarrhea attack?

\_\_\_\_ 4. Do you sometimes have diarrhea? If so, is it severe? \_\_\_\_

If you answered yes to either #3 or 4, do parasite testing at a specialty lab.

## Antibiotic-Sensitive Infections

_____ 5. Has any antibiotic improved your CFS/FMS symptoms?

_____ 6. Do you have scabbing scalp sores?

_____ 7. Do you have chronic respiratory infections/lung congestion?

_____ 8. Do you have chronic or intermittent low-grade fevers?

_____ 9. Do you have chronic vertigo (where it feels like you or the room is spinning in a circle)?

_____ 10. Have you had severe reactions (not including rash, itching, throat swelling, or trouble breathing) to two or more different antibiotics?

_____ 11. Did your illness begin after a tick bite and a bull's-eye rash?

If yes to any of the questions in #5–11, check off #32.


## Viral Infections

_____ 12. Did your CFS/FMS begin with a flu-like infection?

_____ 13. Do you have chronic flu-like symptoms despite being on Cortef (hydrocortisone)?

If yes to either #12 or 13, check off #27 and 31.


## An Ounce of Prevention . . . (for Everyone)

_____ 14. Would you like something to keep on hand for treating acute respiratory infections?

If yes, check off #29 and 30 to keep in your medicine cabinet.

# 7.

# N—Nutrition: Optimizing Your Body's Ability to Heal, Including Ribose, a Powerful New Nutrient

For those of you who watch what you eat, here's the final word on nutrition and health. It's a relief to know the truth after all those conflicting medical studies:

1. The Japanese eat very little fat and drink very little red wine, and they suffer fewer heart attacks than Americans.
2. The French eat lots of fatty cheese and rich food and drink lots of wine, and they suffer fewer heart attacks than Americans.
3. The Italians drink a lot of red wine and eat lots of carbohydrate-rich pasta, and they suffer fewer heart attacks than Americans.
4. The Germans drink a lot of beer and eat lots of sausages and fats, and they suffer fewer heart attacks than Americans.

**Conclusion:** Eat and drink what you like. Speaking English is apparently what kills you.

There are so many medical myths floating around that it's a wonder anybody can enjoy their food anymore. So here are today's nutrition "Myth Busters":

1. Eggs are bad for you and raise cholesterol. Busted and busted again! Over six studies have shown that eating six eggs a day for six weeks has no effect on cholesterol. In fact, eggs are the healthiest protein you can get short of eating another human being. So enjoy!
2. Salt is bad for you. Busted! Studies show that people who eat the so-called recommended amount of salt die younger than those who eat more. Especially for those with adrenal fatigue, salt restriction is a good way to crash and burn. So enjoy adding salt to your food as your taste directs you.
3. Coffee and tea are bad for you. Busted! These are both natural compounds that are chock-full of healthy antioxidants. The trick is to not overdo the caffeine, so after your first cup or two of regular coffee or tea, switch to decaf.
4. Alcohol is bad for you. Busted! Those who drink up to two drinks a day live longer than teetotalers.

And the list goes on and on. In general, the best way to tell what is good for you is by how it makes you feel in the long term. If overall you feel great, then what you are doing is working. If it gives you great pleasure at the same time, that's an even better sign that it is good for you.

So what is it that's best avoided? Basically, those things that make you feel bad overall. I say overall because some things, such as heroin, make you feel better right away but much worse overall. The food equivalent of this is excess sugar.

This doesn't mean you can't have sugar at all. In fact, eating fruits and dark chocolate is actually very healthy. Simply avoid processed foods that have been loaded with sugar to cover the taste of "food-like materials" that are rancid or gross. Save your sugar budget for dessert, where it belongs.

Especially important? Cut out sodas and fruit juices that have three-quarters teaspoon of sugar per ounce. This means that forty-eight-ounce "Big Burp" soda at your local Quickie Mart that contains a whopping thirty-six spoonfuls of sugar. It will give you a quick high but leave you crashing overall.

> *Moderation in all things—including moderation.*
> —MARK TWAIN

So my nutrition advice?

1. Eat what makes you feel good.
2. Avoid excess sugar and sweets in processed foods.
3. When convenient, choose whole foods over processed junk. When looking at the ingredients (which is a very good idea), I recommend this simple guideline: "If you can't read it, don't eat it!" Anyway, do you really want to stuff your body with a chemical soup?
4. Drink plenty of water. If your mouth and lips are dry, it means you're thirsty.

# Start with the Basics—a Healthy Diet

Although I strongly recommend taking nutritional supplements to ensure obtaining the necessary nutrients, I want to begin by stressing that a healthy diet is most important. Eat a lot of whole grains, fresh fruits (whole fruit, not fruit juice), and fresh vegetables. Many raw vegetables have enzymes that help boost energy levels. You do not have to cut out all foods that might be bad or eat a diet that is impossible to follow. All you need to do is consume a diet that is reasonably healthy and low in added sugar. The more unprocessed your diet is, the healthier you will be. Your body will tell you what's good for you by making you feel good.

## THE PROBLEM WITH SUGAR

I am not concerned with the sugar normally found in food as in an apple or orange. It is the 140 pounds per person added each year in food processing.

In addition to causing people to lose 18 percent of their vitamins and minerals, the excess sugar also:

1. Suppresses the immune system. The amount of sugar in one can of soda suppresses immune function by 30 percent for three hours.

2. Stimulates yeast overgrowth. Yeast grows by fermenting sugar, and the yeast says thank you for eating sugar by making billions of baby yeasties.

3. Amplifies symptoms of hypoglycemia, such as irritability when

hungry and the associated need for marriage counseling and divorce lawyers (seriously!).

## WANT TO HAVE YOUR CAKE AND EAT IT, TOO?

Start by cutting out the sugary drinks. Sixteen ounces of either soda or fruit juice (yep, that includes "unsweetened" orange and apple juice) packs a whopping twelve teaspoons of sugar. Eat an apple or an orange instead. And enjoy up to an ounce of dark chocolate each day. Though not low-calorie, I consider dark chocolate to be a health food. That's why I tell people, "Avoid sugar—except for chocolate!"

I think pleasure is good for you. So here are some delicious yet healthy sweet things to enjoy:

1. Sugar-free chocolate. Russell Stover has an excellent line available in most supermarkets and drugstores. If you want some sugar-free chocolate to die for, go to www.abdallah candies.com, go to "products," and click on the "sugar-free chocolates" page. For another delicious brand, check out the sugar-free chocolates at the Rocky Mountain Candy Factory (www.rmcf.com).
2. Instead of sodas, Zevia has a whole line of sugar-free sodas that are stevia sweetened. In addition, Vitaminwater and SoBe both have a sugar-free line that is stevia sweetened and all natural. The Vitaminwater Zero Go-Go Mixed Berry even has some ribose in it!

# Nutritional Support

Even if you're eating well, the modern diet is awful, with an average of 18 percent of calories coming from sugar, and another 18 percent from white flour (which is a nutritional wasteland). Then enough fat is added so that half of what we eat consists of "empty calories," which are basically devoid of vitamins and minerals. Because of this, for the first time in human history we are seeing obese people being malnourished!

I will begin by discussing simple nutritional support to help supply the nutrients we should be getting from our diet. I will then finish the chapter with a discussion of special energy nutrients that are made by our bodies specifically to make energy.

# Which Nutrient Do I Need?

People often ask me which vitamin or nutrient they need.

The answer? All of them!

Fortunately, this is a lot easier than it sounds

Whether you have day-to-day fatigue, or CFS/FMS, optimizing nutritional supplementation can dramatically improve how you feel. Here's how to make it easy.

## • • • VITAMIN AND MINERAL SUPPLEMENTS • • •

The argument that the average modern American does not need vitamin tablets is simply not valid. One study reported in the *American Journal of Clinical Nutrition* showed that fewer than 5 percent of the study participants consumed the recommended daily amounts (RDAs) of all their needed vitamins and minerals. What is frightening is that this study was conducted on U.S. Department of Agriculture (USDA) research center employees, people who should be especially aware of proper nutrition.

So for those who say that you are "just making expensive urine" by taking a multivitamin (because it goes out in the urine), I recommend they consider what would happen if they stopped drinking water—which also just goes out in their urine!

# Making Nutrient Support Simple

In addition to a healthy diet, it is important to get good nutritional support with supplements. To keep it easy, I recommend the Energy Revitalization System vitamin powder (made by Enzymatic Therapy) or the Daily Energy Enfusion (from Integrative Therapeutics). One simple low-cost drink a day replaces more than thirty-five supplement pills, supplying virtually all of the vitamins and minerals you should be getting from your diet (the exceptions being iron, potassium, and essential fatty acids). I did help create these products; however, as noted above, my royalties are donated to charity.

I lecture frequently to hundreds of the world's leading nutritional experts at their annual conferences, and I regularly put out the challenge that if any of them can get what's in the one drink in less than thirty-five capsules, I'd give them fifty dollars. No one has managed to do it yet, and these are the experts. Try it yourself. It usually takes fifty-plus capsules (see Appendix E, "Other Resources," for further information).

Because the Energy Revitalization System is a powder, it can be taken many ways. Some like to add it to plain yogurt. Others add the orange-flavored form (my wife's favorite) to two ounces of orange juice, two ounces of water, and four ounces of milk so that it tastes like an orange smoothie. Others like the berry flavor (my favorite) and simply stir it in water to avoid the sugar in fruit juices. If hand-mixing it instead of using a blender, the best way to mix powders is to put the powder in a dry glass, add two to three ounces of whatever liquid you're using, give it a few stirs till any lumps are gone, and then add the rest of the liquid. It's the most worthwhile thirty seconds you'll spend each day!

The main side effects caused by multivitamins that give optimal nutritional support are gas, diarrhea, or an upset stomach, which occur in a small percentage of people. If this is a problem, simply take one half scoop a day instead of the whole scoop. For most people, that is plenty, and it also cuts the cost in half. So simply adjust the powder dose to what feels best to you.

It is helpful to know that any supplement containing B vitamins will turn your urine bright yellow. This is normal and simply shows that you are absorbing the B vitamins well. They come out in the urine *after* they're finished doing their job. The vitamin powder is excellent for anybody who would like an outstanding multivitamin, and the Energy Revitalization System vitamin powder is available in most health food stores or at www.endfatigue.com.

The vitamin powder includes optimal levels of each of the vitamins, minerals, energy cofactors, and amino acids that you should be getting from your diet. Information on why each nutrient is so critical can be found in the "Nutrition Guide" at www.vitality101.com, in the long version of *From Fatigued to Fantastic!*, or on the free iPhone and Android app Cures A-Z.

So overall, aim to eat whole foods instead of junk, avoid excess sugar, drink plenty of water (or other sugar-free beverages), and take the Energy Revitalization System vitamin powder. I add a 5-gram scoop of ribose (Corvalen, discussed later in this chapter) to the vitamin powder each morning to turbocharge my energy.

Let's take a moment to look at a few other nutrients that can be very helpful in addition to what's in the vitamin powder. We will begin by discussing deficiencies of nutrients that should be in our food. We will then finish with a discussion of special nutrients made by our body, which can be dramatically effective at increasing energy.

## THE IMPORTANCE OF VITAMIN B$_{12}$

Some people have trouble absorbing vitamin B$_{12}$, and getting it into the brain where it is critically needed. Because of this, we have a very high amount of vitamin B$_{12}$ in the vitamin powder (500 µg). Some people with CFS/FMS benefit from even higher levels by injection. If a person's vitamin B$_{12}$ level is under 540 pg/ml ("normal" is anything over 200, which is absurd), your doctor may want to start treatment with a 1 cc (1,000- to 3,000+-microgram) injection one to five times a week, giving at least fifteen total injections. These shots are safe and fairly inexpensive.

## NAC

If you use acetaminophen frequently, you should also take 500 to 1,000 milligrams of supplemental N-Acetyl-L-Cysteine (NAC) each day so you don't deplete your glutathione levels. I consider taking 650 milligrams a day for three months to be helpful for anyone with CFS/FMS but not day-to-day fatigue. The vitamin powder has 250 mg of NAC.

## IRON

Iron is important because an iron level that is too low can cause fatigue, poor immune function, cold intolerance, restless leg syndrome, decreased thyroid function, and poor memory. I routinely recommend that all my chronic fatigue patients have their iron level checked by doing a blood test called a ferritin level. Technically, this is normal if it is over 12, a level that misses over 90 percent of people with severe iron deficiency anemia. So once again, ignore the "normal range" and aim to get your ferritin level up over 60 ng/ml.

If your ferritin is elevated, which can also cause fibromyalgia, your doctor should determine whether you have a genetic disease of excess iron called hemochromatosis. If caught early, it is laughably easy to treat. If caught late, after causing diabetes and liver failure, it can kill you.

Although cosmetic issues may seem small relative to the debilitating nature of CFS, they are still important, as few of us would be happy with the severe hair thinning often seen in CFS/FMS. Iron deficiency contributes to hair loss and, according to Cleveland Clinic dermatologists, treatment of iron deficiency is important for restoring hair growth. In their opinion, "treatment for hair loss is enhanced when iron deficiency, with or without anemia, is treated." They aim to keep the ferritin level over 70 ng/ml, but not higher than 150, as too much iron can also be toxic, so if taking iron, it's good to keep an eye on the blood levels. Low thyroid and simply the stress of the CFS/FMS can also contribute to hair loss. When these are treated, most often hair growth resumes after nine months.

Iron must be taken on an empty stomach; otherwise you will lose 85 percent of the absorption. Do not take calcium or iron supplements within six hours of your thyroid dose, as they block thyroid absorption. It is normal for iron to cause constipation and a black stool. Fortunately, if you take the iron every other day, you get almost as much benefit as taking it daily—with lower side effects. If the ferritin level is under 60 ng/ml, I give 30 to 60 milligrams of iron a day, making sure that the supplement also has at least 60 milligrams of vitamin C to enhance absorption. For those who cannot tolerate iron because of upset stomach or constipation, Floradix makes a liquid iron supplement that has 11 milligrams of iron per dose, is well absorbed, and does not upset the stomach.

A final note on iron: Ferritin levels that are elevated, especially if the iron percent saturation test is also over 45 percent, can be dangerous, and may reflect a genetic disease called hemochromatosis. Again, if caught early, it is very easy to treat, but can kill you if missed. So be sure your physician addresses this if your ferritin level is elevated!

## FISH OILS

The two key omega-3 essential fatty acids in fish oil are eicosapentaenoic acid (EPA) and docosahexaenoic acid (DHA), the latter being a major component of brain tissue. Perhaps the old wives' tales were right in calling fish "brain food."

Fish-oil essential fatty acid levels are often low in CFS/FMS and research shows that supplementation improves symptoms. Even in healthy people, fish-oil supplements decrease depression and inflammation.

The best way to get these essential fatty acids is by eating three to four servings of a fatty fish each week such as salmon, tuna, or sardines (fried fish does not count). It is also reasonable to supplement with essential fatty acids, and it is part of my daily regimen along with the vitamin powder and ribose. Most brands require taking eight to sixteen fish-oil capsules a day, resulting not only in their being irritating and high cost, but also in creating "fish-oil burps." I like cats as much as the next guy, but having them follow me around all day waiting for me to burp got annoying. The good news? Research has shown that a new way to extract the fish-oil essential fatty acids dramatically increases absorption. So all you need is one tablet a day of Vectomega (by EuroPharma) instead of eight a day of most fish oils! Out of thousands of natural products added each year, it won the best new product of the year award!

## OTHER NUTRITIONAL TIPS FOR CFS/FMS

Most people with fibromyalgia find that they feel best with a high-protein, low-carbohydrate diet. In addition, add as much salt to your food as your body wants (except sometimes in high blood pressure or heart failure), as salt restriction in the presence of an underactive adrenal will make people crash and burn. But diet is also not a "one size fits all" prescription. Everybody is different, so check to see what diet leaves your body feeling the best overall.

People with CFS/FMS often ask if they are allowed to drink alcohol. I tell them yes as long as it doesn't make them feel worse. Some people with CFS/FMS, especially when candida is severe, feel lousy when they have any alcohol. In these cases I don't have to tell them not to drink, as their body has already done so. For everyone else, up to two drinks a day is okay.

Same for caffeine. Caffeine can aggravate symptoms of low blood sugar often seen in those with adrenal fatigue. In those who don't have this problem, one or two cups of tea or coffee a day is okay as long as it is not taken too late in the afternoon, as it can aggravate insomnia. The problem is when people start using the caffeine as an "energy loan shark," drinking four or more cups a day to function. That's when it actually starts to drag you down.

## WHY DO PEOPLE WITH CFS AND FIBROMYALGIA NEED MORE NUTRITIONAL SUPPORT THAN EVERYBODY ELSE?

In addition to eating the Standard American Diet (often appropriately abbreviated as SAD), with half of its calories being stripped of nutrients, people with CFS/FMS have additional problems:

1. They crave sugar more than most people because of the low adrenal, candida, and increased thirst (what I call "drink like a fish, pee like a racehorse" syndrome).
2. Because of increased bowel infections, people with CFS/FMS have decreased nutrient absorption.
3. Because of the illness they have increased nutrient needs, such as $B_{12}$, magnesium, iron, essential fatty acids, and other nutrients.

# Special Nutrients for Everyone with Fatigue

There are several critical specialized nutrients that can powerfully boost energy production and that are not in the vitamin powder, such as ribose, coenzyme $Q_{10}$, and acetyl-L-carnitine. These three do not reflect nutritional deficiencies but rather increased needs for optimizing energy production. These often can be stopped after four to nine months, although many people choose to take them for the long term as well (especially the ribose).

So let's jump-start our energy production and set ourselves up for success.

# Jump-Starting Your Body's Energy Furnaces

Each cell in your body contains structures called mitochondria, the tiny furnaces in each cell that produce energy by burning calories. Many problems, including some viral infections, can suppress these, so it is critical to go to the heart of the problem and optimize our body's energy furnaces. So let's begin our discussion with nutritional support that directly increases energy production.

# The Role of Energy Production

It used to be that for people with day-to-day fatigue, simply taking a couple of days vacation or rest, catching up on sleep, and eating well was enough for them to rebuild energy stores. Unfortunately, it seems that more often than not, this is no longer the case. So whether you simply are suffering from the fatigue of modern life or the severe energy deficiencies seen in CFS and fibromyalgia, let's begin with ways to turbocharge your energy production. We simply can't overcome fatigue if the cells and tissues in our bodies don't have enough energy.

## THE CONSEQUENCES OF SEVERE MITOCHONDRIAL DYSFUNCTION

People with fibromyalgia and CFS have almost 20 percent less energy in their muscles than normal, and they have trouble using oxygen effectively to make energy. To get an idea of what this means, think of taking a 20 percent pay cut. Ouch! A large number of clinical findings common in CFS/FMS can be explained by mitochondrial furnace malfunction:

*Hypothalamic suppression.* Particularly severe changes in the hypothalamus have been seen in genetic mitochondrial dysfunction syndromes.

*Brain fog.* Mitochondrial dysfunction can cause decreases in levels of neurotransmitters in the brain, specifically low dopamine and acetylcholine, and possibly low serotonin.

*Sensitivities and allergies.* Decreased ability of the liver to eliminate toxins and medications could also contribute to sensitivities to medications and environmental factors, as well as food sensitivities.

*Postexertion fatigue.* Low energy production and accumulation of excessive amounts of lactic acid in muscles could inhibit recovery after exercise.

*Poor digestion.* Mitochondrial dysfunction could also contribute to bowel-related problems along with the lack of digestive enzymes and buildup of unhealthy gut infections.

*Heart dysfunction.* Research shows a decrease in heart function in CFS and fibromyalgia, which also contributes to the

> symptoms. This is not caused by a problem with the heart itself but rather with its energy production.
>
> Thus, mitochondrial dysfunction might well be the root cause—or at least a contributing factor—of many of the problems seen in CFS/FMS.

# Improving Mitochondrial Function

A key question is whether anything can be done to make your cellular energy furnaces work better. Fortunately, the answer is a resounding yes! Several natural treatments are available to do just that. Let's begin with D-ribose, a critical key to energy production.

## D-RIBOSE—THE NATURAL BODY ENERGIZER

To understand energy production, it helps to look at critical "energy molecules" such as ATP (adenosine triphosphate). These represent the energy currency in your body and are like the paper that money is printed on. You can have all the fuel (calories) you want, but if it cannot be converted to these molecules, it is useless—and simply gets turned into fat.

B vitamins are a key component of many of these molecules. We find that these are helpful, but it is clear that other key components are missing. In looking at the biochemistry of these energy molecules, we saw that they were also made of two other key components—

adenine and ribose. Adenine (which used to be called vitamin B$_4$) is plentiful in the body, so we turned our attention to ribose, which is made in your body in a slow, laborious process. We found that ribose is low in energy-deficient states, making it hard to get your furnaces working again even after the other underlying problems were treated.

This was like one of those "Eureka!" moments, when things come together. Not having ribose would be like trying to build a fire without kindling—nothing would happen. We wondered if giving ribose to people with CFS/FMS, one of the worst energy deficiencies in the world, would jump-start their energy furnaces. I am lead author on two studies looking at this question, and the results amazed us!

The two studies included almost 300 people with CFS and fibromyalgia at fifty-four different clinics. Ribose was given at a dose of 5 grams three times a day for three weeks. People reported their energy increased an average of about 60 percent by three weeks. In addition, mental clarity, sleep, and overall well-being improved significantly while pain levels dropped. The abstracts of our most recent study can be seen in Appendix B.

Ribose is available over the counter and is one of the few natural products that actually started with physicians and then moved into health food stores.

It is critical to use the proper dose, which is 5 grams (5,000 milligrams) three times a day for the first three weeks. It can then be dropped to twice a day. I recommend the Corvalen form of ribose, as it is high quality and is packaged with a 5-gram dosing scoop in it. One 280-gram container will be enough to tell you if it will work. Corvalen M (which has ribose plus magnesium and malic acid) is also available, but if you are also taking the Energy Revitalization System vitamin powder (see page 159), you are already getting the magnesium and malic acid, and the regular Corvalen is more cost-effective.

Let's look at ribose in more detail to see what it does.

## D-RIBOSE ACCELERATES ENERGY RECOVERY

D-ribose (which is what I am referring to when I say ribose) is a simple five-carbon sugar (known as a pentose by biochemists) that is found naturally in our bodies. But ribose is not like other toxic sugars, such as table sugar (sucrose), corn sugar (glucose), and fructose. When we consume ribose, the body recognizes that it is different from other sugars and preserves it for the vital work of actually making the energy molecules that power the heart, muscles, brain, and every other tissue in the body—making it healthy and helpful even for people who can't tolerate sugar.

The amount of ATP we have in our tissues determines whether we will be fatigued or will have the energy we need to live vital, active lives. Ribose provides the key building block of ATP, and the presence of ribose in the cell stimulates the metabolic pathway our bodies use to actually make this vital compound. If the cell does not have enough ribose, it cannot make ATP. So, when cells and tissues become energy-starved, the availability of ribose is critical to energy recovery.

## THE LINK BETWEEN RIBOSE, ENERGY, AND FATIGUE

Two very interesting studies in animals showed how dramatic the effect of ribose could be on energy recovery in fatigued muscle. These studies were conducted by Dr. Ron Terjung, one of the top muscle physiologists in the United States. In their research, Dr. Terjung and his coinvestigators found that ribose administration in fatigued muscle increased the rate of energy recovery by 340 to 430 percent, depending on which type of muscle was tested. He also found that even very small amounts of ribose had the effect of helping the muscle cell preserve energy, a process known as energy salvage, and the higher the ribose dose, the more dramatic the effect on energy preservation. Although this groundbreaking research was done in animals, it was instrumental in defining the biochemistry and physiology associated with the use of ribose in overcoming heart and muscle fatigue in humans. But most of us with CFS and FMS are neither top athletes nor animals, so the question most of us wanted explained remained unanswered: "How will ribose affect me?"

Research in ribose and CFS/FMS began with a case study that was published in the prestigious journal *Pharmacotherapy* in 2004. This case study told the story of a veterinary surgeon diagnosed with fibromyalgia. For months, this dedicated doctor found herself becoming more and more fatigued, with pain becoming so profound that she was finally unable to stand during surgery. As a result, she was forced to all but give up the practice she loved.

Upon hearing that a clinical study on ribose in congestive heart failure was under way in the university where she worked, she asked if she could try the ribose to see if it might help her overcome the mind-numbing fatigue she experienced from her disease. After three weeks of ribose therapy, she was back in the operating room, practicing normally, with no muscle pain or stiffness, and without the fatigue that had kept her bedridden for many months.

Being a doctor, she was skeptical, not believing that a simple sugar could have such a dramatic effect on her condition. Within two weeks of stopping the ribose therapy, however, she was out of the operating room and back in bed. So, to again test the theory, she began ribose therapy a second time. The result was similar to her first experience, and she was back doing surgery in days. After yet a third round of stopping (with the return of symptoms) and starting the ribose therapy (with the reduction of symptoms), she was convinced, and she has been on ribose therapy since that time. This was the start of countless numbers of people around the world getting their life back with ribose.

Ribose regulates how much energy we have in our bodies, and for those suffering from fatigue, muscle soreness, stiffness, and a host of related medical complications, the relief found in energy restoration can be life changing. This is why I recommend that people with fatigue begin with 5 grams of D-ribose (one scoop of Corvalen) three times a day for two to three weeks, then twice a day. For those with day-to-day fatigue, simply adding a 5-gram scoop to your morning vitamin powder each day may be plenty.

Most people feel the difference by the end of a single 280-gram container of ribose (Corvalen). The few who don't may retry it twelve to sixteen weeks into the other treatments we discuss. You'll be glad you did.

Interestingly, one of our study patients had an abnormal heart rhythm called atrial fibrillation. Ribose is outstanding in the treatment of heart disease as well because it restores energy production in the heart muscle. Because of this, it was not surprising that this man's atrial fibrillation also went away with the ribose treatment, and he was able to stop his heart medications as well. It is common that people with even crippling heart disease feel dramatically better after six weeks on ribose. If you know anybody with heart disease, have them use the recipe below. After six weeks, they will often have their life back!

## A RECIPE FOR HEALING HEART DISEASE

Heart disease is a common cause of fatigue. Whether the problem is heart failure, angina, or abnormal heart rhythms, increasing heart muscle efficiency can result in remarkable improvement clinically. It can also be lifesaving.

Ribose—Take 5 grams three times a day for six weeks, then twice a day.

Coenzyme $Q_{10}$—Take 200 milligrams a day.

Energy Revitalization System vitamin powder—one half to one scoop a day.

Acetyl-L-carnitine—500 milligrams three times a day for six weeks, then 500 milligrams a day.

In severe cases, add the herb hawthorn along with magnesium orotate—3,000 milligrams a day.

Use the above with the okay of your holistic physician. Two cautions: people taking the blood thinner Coumadin *must* get their physician's okay before adding any supplement or medication, and magnesium must be used cautiously in those with kidney failure.

# Other Key Energy Nutrients

Although ribose is the most promising energy nutrient, others are also worth looking at. Most of these only need to be taken for four to nine months, though some people choose to take them longer. I personally take my ribose and coenzyme $Q_{10}$ every day, even though I feel great. It makes me feel even better! You will know whether to keep taking them by how you feel.

Other key energy boosters include:

*Coenzyme $Q_{10}$.* Coenzyme $Q_{10}$, 200 milligrams a day. I recommend the Smart $Q_{10}$ by Enzymatic Therapy as it contains vitamin E to increase absorption. A special note: most cholesterol-lowering drugs deplete coenzyme $Q_{10}$ and in my experience can cause and worsen fatigue and pain. Anyone taking cholesterol-lowering medications (called statins) should also take 200 milligrams a day of coenzyme $Q_{10}$.

*Malic acid.* This is needed to "rescue" part of the key energy producer in the body called the Krebs energy cycle. Malic acid is a compound that occurs naturally in foods, in fruits in general, and in especially high levels in apples. (Remember the old saying: An apple a day keeps the doctor away.) Malic acid and magnesium can easily be found in good vitamin powders, such as the Energy Revitalization System.

*Acetyl-L-carnitine.* This is not needed in day-to-day fatigue but is important if you have CFS or fibromyalgia, where muscle biopsies show that it is routinely deficient. Carnitine is found in animal flesh (think "carni-vore"), and any brand is fine as long as it is pure acetyl-L-carnitine. Although you may not see a marked effect, in CFS/FMS it helps lay the foundation for your getting better and may even help you lose some of the weight you have gained. Take 500 milligrams twice a day for four months.

So, to summarize, the mitochondria are the energy furnaces in your cells that burn food for energy. To get these mitochondrial energy furnaces turbocharged:

1. Take a good multivitamin powder like the Energy Revitalization System.
2. Take D-ribose (Corvalen), 5,000 milligrams three times a day for three weeks, then two times a day in CFS/FMS or once each morning for day-to-day fatigue. It's a powder that looks and tastes like sugar and does not act as food for yeast. It can be added to food or drinks, even hot tea.
3. Take 200 milligrams of coenzyme $Q_{10}$ daily for four months (I prefer chewable wafers that include a bit of vitamin E to help absorption such as Smart $Q_{10}$ by Enzymatic Therapy).

I would recommend these three for everyone with fatigue, or even if you simply would like more energy, and I'd take them for the long term (this is what I still take daily). If the cost is not prohibitive, add acetyl-L-carnitine, 500 milligrams three to four times a day for three to four months.

## INTRAVENOUS NUTRITIONAL THERAPIES

A very powerfully effective treatment that I have found for treating chronic fatigue syndrome and fibromyalgia is the use of intravenous (IV) nutritional support. Especially important is the magnesium, which when given via IV opens up blood vessels to tight muscles, flooding these starved areas with nutrients and washing away the toxins. You'll find that when your holistic doctor administers these injections, you'll feel a warm flush in the areas that have been most significantly affected by your illness.

I recommend that, if possible, all patients with CFS/FMS receive these IV therapies at least once a week for six weeks and then as needed. Along with ribose and the other supplements I've recommended (which should be continued while on the IVs), the IV therapies can dramatically "jump-start" some of your body's systems and can markedly shorten the time it takes to begin feeling better. Many physicians refer to these therapies as Myers' cocktails. If you have a physician who is willing to give nutritional IVs, I strongly recommend that you have them.

## Important Points

Eat whole foods instead of processed foods whenever it's convenient.

Remove *excess* caffeine from your diet.

Remove sugar and other sweeteners from your diet. Stevia, a sweet-tasting herb, and even saccharin and Sweet'N Low (I do not recommend aspartame) can be used as substitutes. They taste good and stevia is healthy.

Increase water intake so that your lips and mouth are not dry. When available, use a high-quality water filter (e.g., Multipure; see www.jacobsonhealth.com or call 410-224-4877). Overall, tap water is better than dehydration or bottled water.

Take one half to one scoop of the Energy Revitalization System multivitamin powder by Enzymatic Therapy daily. This has more than fifty key nutrients in one drink and replaces more than thirty-five capsules of supplements. It is available in most health food stores and at www.endfatigue.com.

Take a 5-gram scoop of ribose (Corvalen) three times a day for three to six weeks and then twice a day for CFS/FMS. For day-to-day fatigue, simply add a 5-gram scoop of ribose to the vitamin powder each morning to turbocharge healthy energy production.

Treat a too-low iron level with an iron supplement. If you have dry eyes, dry mouth, depression, or inflammation, take fish oil (Vecto-mega supplies all you need in one tablet a day).

If you are on cholesterol medications (called statins) or have severe fatigue, add coenzyme $Q_{10}$. Take 200 milligrams a day.

## Questionnaire

(Check off treatments in Appendix C, "Your SHINE Treatment Worksheet.")

_____ 1. Do you have fatigue, CFS/FMS, or pain? Check off #1, 2, and 3—the vitamin powder and ribose offer awesome multi-vitamin and nutritional support for almost everyone.

_____ 2. Do you also have CFS/FMS? If yes, check off #7.

_____ 3. Do you have dry eyes or dry mouth?

_____ 4. Do you have depression or inflammatory problems? If yes to #3 or #4, take fish-oil support; check off #4.

_____ 5. Is your blood ferritin under 60? If yes, check off #5—iron.

_____ 6. Do you have frequent infections or do you use Tylenol often? If yes to either, check off #6—NAC.

# 8.

# E—Exercise, as Able

*I*f *exercise were a pill, everyone would take it.*

That's because exercise can effectively help prevent or treat just about *every* health problem out there, and is critical for optimizing vitality. Because our body has a "use it or lose it" approach to efficiency, the more exercise you do, the better conditioned your body will be—and more energy you will have.

The need for exercise is pretty obvious, so mostly I'm going to focus on some simple tips to make exercising easier. Let's start with the basic rules.

## Rule #1

## Enjoy Your Exercise!
## (Or You Won't Stay with It)

*No pain, no gain.*

You've heard that slogan, of course. It reflects the belief that unless exercise *hurts*, it's not doing its job.

I have another slogan I want you to say to yourself instead.

*Pain is insane!*

Alternatively, "No pain, no gain" is stupid! Pain is your body's way of telling you, "Don't do that." Exercise should be virtually pain-free. And fun-filled.

# Rule #2

# A Little Bit Can Go a Long Way

A common exercise error: you start a new exercise program by doing way too much, way too soon.

People who do this usually *stop* exercising fairly quickly as well—because they hurt!

The body likes *gradual* change, so it can easily and comfortably adapt to new situations.

So remember: a little movement is better than no movement at all.

# Rule #3

# Find an Exercise You Enjoy

Find an activity *you* love to do, look forward to, and that fits into your routine.

Whether you're doing a dance class, going for a walk in the park, doing yoga, or even shopping, doing something you love makes it more likely that you'll stick with it.

# Rule #4

## Have a Regular Scheduled Routine

Meet with a friend to do the exercise. The obligation of meeting somebody means that you're also more likely to show up.

# The Pedometer:
## Your Low-Cost Fitness Coach

It is not necessary to push for high intensity. It's better to simply aim to walk 6,000 to 10,000 steps a day (this is around three to five miles). Walking is a great exercise, especially if done outdoors in the sunshine. Meanwhile, the pedometer will motivate you to do things like park at the far end of the parking lot or take the steps instead of the elevator in order to meet your fitness goal.

It also is enlightening to see where you're starting from. When I first put on a pedometer and then excitedly checked it at the end of the day, it showed I had taken a whopping 687 steps for the whole day! This got me off the couch and out on the walking trail. By taking a half hour and doing a quick two- to three-mile walk, this added 4,000 to 6,000 steps on the pedometer—leaving me a whole lot less embarrassed.

Bottom line: pedometers show you exactly how much you're walking so you get instant feedback and can set a goal to walk more.

## • • • BUYING AND USING A PEDOMETER • • •

1. Choose a pedometer in the fifteen-dollar to twenty-dollar range, which is likely to be accurate.
2. *Wear it in the right spot.* That's on your waistband or belt, two to six inches on either side of your belly button.
3. *Add steps until fit.* Our pedometer experts recommended this strategy for starting to use your pedometer:
   A. Wear the pedometer for three days.
   B. The following week, increase your baseline by 1,000 steps per day.
   C. Add fifty steps a day until you meet your goal. Make this goal the number of steps you *enjoy* walking, even if that is 6,000 steps, and not how many you think you should do.
4. *Add more steps.*
   A. The best way to add a lot more steps to your day: go for a walk. Research also shows that walking with a friend—or a couple of friends—is one of the best ways to use a pedometer.

According to Dr. Caroline Richardson, a research scientist at the VA Medical Center in Ann Arbor, Michigan, "If you give a person a pedometer and tell her to walk 10,000 steps a day, but nobody knows she has a pedometer, and she doesn't know anybody with a pedometer—chances are good she'll throw the thing in a drawer after a week and never look at it again. But if you give everybody in the office a pedometer, and there's a chart on the wall recording each person's progress, and every day people are comparing their step counts and planning a walk at lunch—chances are very good that in a year she'll *still* be using the pedometer. Social support and group activity has an effect on *any* kind of physical activity, and it seems to make a huge difference for pedometer-based walking."

# Exercise and Reconditioning During CFS/Fibromyalgia Treatment

Let's finish up the SHINE intensive care protocol with exercise—*as able*. The key words here are "as able"! Although exercise seems a simple topic to discuss, I know for many of you it has been a difficult one to implement. "Postexertional fatigue" is a common part of CFS/FMS, but it doesn't even begin to express what you have experienced. Postexertional fatigue means that people may feel bedridden for several days after exercise. Meanwhile, some idiots out there still imply to your physician that this isn't a real disease, encouraging them to just tell people to exercise more. I know sometimes it makes you feel like screaming.

But here's the simple truth.

When being treated for any debilitating illness, including cancer-related fatigue, reconditioning is a critical part of getting well. The difference is that no researcher who studies treating cancer-related fatigue with exercise is idiotic enough to imply that this means the cancer is not real. Meanwhile, the postexertional fatigue is fairly unique to CFS/FMS. So that's the difference.

Fortunately, even most researchers looking at exercise therapy in

CFS and fibromyalgia recognize that this is a real and severe illness. And it's okay to simply ignore the ones who don't.

So let's get to what you need to know, so you can recondition despite your CFS/FMS. Because of the body-wide "energy crisis" seen in CFS/FMS, most of you have found that you were unable to condition beyond a certain point (it takes energy to store energy in muscles, which is what conditioning is). Instead, the doctor would push you to exercise, and you would spend the next two days in bed feeling like you had been hit by a truck!

The good news is that as you do SHINE, you will find that your body starts making the energy needed to condition. You will then be able to exercise more and more—and it will actually leave you feeling better and stronger.

For most fibromyalgia patients, the words "exercise as able" do *not* mean starting with jogging or going to the gym. Instead, doable exercises include walking, gentle yoga, and tai chi, to name just a few. For those too ill to do the above, beginning to recondition in a warm-water pool may allow you to begin a walking program after a while.

The key to a successful exercise program is not to overdo it. As Lisa Davenport, an excellent fibromyalgia advocate, tells people, "Get yourself a pedometer, a good pair of walking shoes, a yoga mat, and a positive attitude. Start slowly and take one day at a time. Increase the intensity and duration of your program with caution. Every day will not be the same. Record your accomplishments in a journal and be proud. You will be pleasantly surprised at the number of steps you can accomplish and the increase you will see in your strength and flexibility. Self-empowerment is all you need to get started."

I'd like to thank Lisa for reminding me of the importance of reconditioning as people get well from fibromyalgia. I used to call this the SHIN protocol. Lisa added the "E" for Exercise, to make it SHINE!

Here are a few tips to help you get started:

1. Begin with light exercise like walking or even warm-water walking (in a heated pool) if regular walking is too difficult.

2. Walk to the degree that you feel "good tired" afterward and better the next day. If you feel worse the next day, stop for a few days and then cut back.

3. Walk only as much as you know you comfortably can (or start with five minutes). Then increase by one minute every other day as is comfortable. When you get to a point that leaves you feeling worse the next day, cut back a bit to a comfortable level and continue that amount of walking each day.

4. After ten weeks on the SHINE protocol, your energy production will usually improve considerably, and you'll be able to continue to increase your walking by one minute every other day.

5. When you get to one hour a day, you can increase the intensity of the exercise. Again, listen to your body and only do what feels good to you. You'll know the difference between how "good pain" feels versus "bad pain" or crashing. Overall, *"No pain, no gain"* is stupid. Pain is your body's way of saying "Don't do that!"

6. *Do* consider a pedometer. It makes it more fun to be able to see your endurance go up (set it for total steps you walk a day). You may not notice an extra fifty steps a day without it. But increasing by fifty steps a day will get people up to the magic 6,000 to

10,000 steps a day in six months. And this isn't just an excellent level for fibromyalgia. It is an excellent level for anyone, as it equals three to five miles a day!

7. Unless it is cold, and the cold flares your pain, I recommend you get your exercise by walking outside, so you can get sunshine—your key source of vitamin D. Many people with CFS/FMS, or chronic pain in general, are vitamin D deficient. Vitamin D from sunshine (or supplements) will help improve immune function and will also decrease the risk of hypertension, diabetes, and cancer (low vitamin D contributes to over 85,000 cancer deaths a year in the United States).

8. When it's cold outside, wear woolen long underwear. A cold breeze can throw muscles into spasm. So can sweating during the walk if you're overdressed. Woolen long johns will soak up any sweat and wick it away from your skin. Meanwhile, don't forget a scarf and hat. More info on this in chapter 9—"Pain Relief."

Even without fibromyalgia, anybody put on bed rest will decondition very quickly. This happens even to extremely fit astronauts when they go into a weightless environment for a few weeks. So even though overdoing it has taught you hard lessons, the magic balance can leave you conditioned without crashing.

And remember: as you do the SHINE protocol, energy production will increase, allowing you to condition.

You now have learned the basics of the SHINE protocol and know the keys that you need in order to recover.

Welcome to getting your life back!

# Important Points

Find a way to exercise that feels good. Do it with a friend on a regular schedule.

Get a pedometer and slowly increase the lengths of your walks as feels best, aiming for 6,000 to 10,000 steps a day. Take your time reaching this goal—there is no hurry!

If you have CFS/FMS, the key is to exercise *as able*, because if you overdo it, you will be wiped out the next few days.

# PART 3

# Pain Relief and Other Health Issues

# 9.

# Natural and Prescription
# Pain Relief

Whether you have day-to-day pain from arthritis, muscle pains, headaches, or other causes, or the widespread and often severe pain of fibromyalgia, relief is available. As noted earlier, *treating the underlying cause of the pain*, by addressing sleep loss, hormonal dysfunctions, underlying infections, nutritional deficiencies, and maintaining flexibility with exercise can get rid of many pains, especially muscle and fibromyalgia pain. This takes time, and during that period it is not acceptable to leave people in pain. Unfortunately, in some cases we also cannot yet get to the underlying cause of the pain. Either way, it is simply not acceptable to be left in pain, and I have found in treating thousands of chronic pain patients that almost everybody can get excellent pain relief. Unfortunately, most physicians are simply not trained in pain management, resulting in one out of four adult Americans having inadequately treated pain.

Unfortunately, the one pain treatment that most physicians are taught about is to give arthritis medications like Motrin or Celebrex (called NSAIDs, nonsteroidal anti-inflammatory drugs). In addition to not helping fibromyalgia or muscle pain, research shows that these medications unnecessarily kill over 30,000 Americans a year, causing 16,500 deaths a year from bleeding ulcers while doubling to tripling the risk of heart attack and stroke.

Fortunately, there are much better ways to get pain relief. If your physician doesn't know how to safely and effectively get you pain free, it doesn't mean you need to live with the pain. It just means that you need to find a pain or fibromyalgia specialist who knows how to treat your pain, and most of you can get pain free simply by using the information in this book!

Let's start with some very safe and powerfully effective natural therapies.

# Natural Pain Treatments

Many natural treatments can dramatically relieve pain. They can be used in combination with pain medications as well.

## HERBAL TREATMENTS

There are two herbal mixes that are outstanding for pain in general, including fibromyalgia pain. The first is a mix of willow bark, boswellia, and cherry called End Pain by Enzymatic Therapy. They can also be found in the mix called Pain Formula by Integrative Therapeutics. The second is an herbal mix called Curamin, by Euro-Pharma. This rather outstanding pain-relief product is a mix of a special, highly absorbed curcumin (called BCM 95), boswellia, DLPA (DL phenylalanine), and nattokinase.

Let's look at each of these components.

*Willow bark* is the original source of aspirin but is much more effective than aspirin and without the toxicity. In head-on studies, willow bark was twice as effective as Motrin for chronic lower-back pain. When before and after endoscopy was done, looking down into the stomach, the willow bark caused no stomach-lining irritation, whereas ibuprofen caused severe gastritis.

*Boswellia* is another name for the old biblical herb frankincense. It seems that the three wise men knew what they were doing, as studies have shown that boswellia drops arthritis pain as much as a dramatic 90 percent. Boswellia also helps with many kinds of inflammation beyond arthritis, including colitis and asthma.

*Curcumin*, which comes from turmeric, is the yellow spice in Indian food such as curry. There have been over 1,000 studies done on the spice showing dramatic benefits for pain relief, inflammation, and even the treatment and prevention of cancer and Alzheimer's. The problem has been that it is so poorly absorbed that one had to essentially be living on Indian food to get enough to be meaningful. This changed dramatically when it was discovered that adding the essential oils back in, as is done in a special product called BCM 95, increased absorption by almost 700 percent. This meant that one capsule could now do what seven of the next best used to do.

*DL phenylalanine (DLPA)* is an amino acid that increases levels of your body's own natural painkillers called endorphins and dopamine. *Nattokinase* helps break down inflammation, allowing the herbs to get to the areas they need to in order to speed healing. These two herbal mixes have been outstanding for pain in general. In fact, a recent head-on study comparing a mix of boswellia and the special curcumin above (called Healthy Knees and Joints by EuroPharma) to Celebrex found the herbs to be dramatically more effective for arthritis. Meanwhile, Curamin has often been helpful in easing pain, even among people whom no medications, including morphine, had helped. I call it "a pain relief miracle!"

Additional effective treatments for arthritis pain include glucosamine sulfate 750 milligrams twice a day, chondroitin 400 milligrams twice a day, and MSM (methylsulfonylmethane) 2,500 milligrams a day. All of these plus the herbal mixes above can be used together for three months along with arthritis medications. At that time, most people find that their arthritis has either gone away or settled down dramatically. I then wean my patients off their arthritis medications, and then wean off one of the natural therapies each two weeks as able. The natural therapies can then be used as needed. Interestingly, research shows that arthritis is kind of like a fire. It takes six to twelve weeks to put it out, but whether on the natural therapies or prescription medications, after three months the pain often stays gone and the treatments can be taken simply on an as-needed basis.

Let's move on to fibromyalgia pain, but those of you who have other pain issues may want to read this section as well: what we discuss is very effective for many kinds of pain. In addition, I invite you to read my book *Pain Free 1-2-3*, which goes through each kind of pain and how to eliminate it.

# Pain—Intensive Care for Fibromyalgia

## General Pain Relief
## for Fibromyalgia—Natural

Here is a good way to start:

1. Begin naturally with the End Pain and/or Curamin herbal mixes, taking one or two tablets of each three times a day. Benefits are often seen in thirty to sixty minutes, but for chronic pain take it for six weeks to see the full effect. At that time, the dose can be reduced to the level needed to maintain relief. These natural therapies can be combined and also taken along with pain medications, increasing their effectiveness and lowering the dose needed. There are also many other natural treatments that can be helpful, including massage, chiropractic, trigger point therapy, yoga, tai chi, qi gong, acupuncture, and a host of others.

2. Treat SHINE to eliminate the root cause of the pain.

    In most cases, fibromyalgia pain is triggered by a lack of energy in the muscles that leads to chronic muscle shortening, stiffness, and pain. Over time, any chronic pain can trigger a secondary nerve pain (neuropathy), as well as what is called central sensitization, where the brain amplifies the pain to get your attention. Because the three new fibromyalgia medications approved by the FDA (Lyrica, Cymbalta, and Savella) work by treating central sensitization, this is what most doctors hear about. But when you treat the underlying causes of the muscle pain with SHINE, the nerve pain and central sensitization often go away.

This was shown in our placebo-controlled study where the SHINE protocol not only improved energy but also dropped pain by 50 percent. Basically, the majority of people in the study no longer qualified as having fibromyalgia by the end of ninety-nine days.

3. Add medications to eliminate pain. Some excellent ones include Neurontin, Ultram, and Skelaxin. These are not only effective but are also cheap (they are generic). If these don't help, I add in Lyrica, Savella, or Cymbalta. All six of these medications can be excellent and give a really good tool kit to get you pain free while you treat the pain's underlying causes.

Let's also look at how to treat a few other types of pain common in CFS/FMS: muscle pain, nerve pain, carpal tunnel syndrome, headaches, and pelvic pain.

# Neuropathy

For nerve pain (can take six to twelve months for the full effect):

1. Take lipoic acid 300 milligrams twice a day along with B vitamins. An excellent mix containing these would be Healthy Feet and Nerves by EuroPharma.
2. Acetyl-L-carnitine 1,500 to 2,000 milligrams a day.

Over time, most people with chronic widespread pain develop nerve pain (called "small fiber neuropathy" or CIDP—Chronic Inflammatory Demyelinating Polyneuropathy). This improves with SHINE, but in severe cases has also been shown to get better with IV gamma globulin infusions (see chapter 6—"Infections: Destroy Your Body's Hidden Invaders").

## HEADACHES

Headaches are very common in fibromyalgia and fall into two main types:

1. *Tension headaches.* These are the most common cause and come from tight muscles. The headaches that occur across your forehead are usually from tight muscles along the side of your neck. These are called the sternocleidomastoid muscles, which turn your head from side to side. If you push down about two inches below the bottom of your earlobe on each side, you can feel the tight marble (called a trigger point) in each muscle, which is the source of the tension headache going across your forehead. The overall treatments for fibromyalgia above will help, but a hot compress or heating pad wrapped around your neck for twenty minutes will also enable these muscles to relax. In addition, using a peppermint/menthol mix topically, such as Tiger Balm, which you can find in any health food store, will help if you rub it on both sides of your forehead (i.e., over the temples). Tension headaches can also be caused by muscles that attach at the base of your skull. These are felt at the top of the head or behind your eyes. A hot compress or heating pad over those tight muscles can also help.

2. *Migraines.* Natural remedies are dramatically effective at preventing migraines, but they take six weeks to start working. Petadolex and IV magnesium can eliminate an acute migraine.

3. *Sinus headaches.* For these, treat the sinusitis caused by candida. This is discussed in chapter 6—"Infections: Destroy Your Body's Hidden Invaders."

## MIGRAINE HEADACHES

These headaches can be very severe and often leave people crippled for days, frequently persisting after a night's sleep (unlike most tension headaches). Migraines are often preceded by an "aura," which may consist of visual disturbances such as flashing lights. Light and sound sensitivity can also be severe.

There is still marked debate over the cause of migraines. For decades, researchers thought that these occurred because of excessive contraction and expansion of the blood vessels in the brain. Others thought that this blood vessel problem occurred because of inadequate serotonin or as a part of the tension headache spectrum. Most likely, it is a common endpoint for many different underlying problems.

### Prevention

1. Take vitamin $B_2$ (riboflavin) 50 to 100 milligrams a day, vitamin $B_{12}$ 500 micrograms a day, and magnesium 200 milligrams a day. All of these can be found in the Energy Revitalization System vitamin powder. For the first six

weeks, add an extra 300 milligrams of vitamin $B_2$. After six weeks this mix drops migraine frequency by over 80 percent.

2. Coenzyme $Q_{10}$—take 200 milligrams a day.
3. If headaches persist after six weeks, do an elimination diet to look for food allergies (see www.vitality101.com and search on "elimination diet").

### Treatment

1. For an acute migraine, take butterbur (called Petadolex) 100 milligrams every two hours for up to three doses until the headache is gone.
2. If in the emergency room, ask for 1 to 2 grams of magnesium given intravenously over fifteen minutes. This eliminates 85 percent of migraines within forty-five minutes, and the migraine will not come back for that episode. It is more effective than Demerol, and the only thing more effective for eliminating an acute migraine is decapitation (not recommended!).

## • • •   ANOTHER CAUSE OF HEADACHE   • • •

A pirate walks into a bar and the bartender says, "Hey, I haven't seen you in a while. You look terrible. What happened?"

"What do you mean?" replies the pirate. "I feel fine."

"What about the wooden leg? You didn't have that before."

"Well, we were in a battle and I got hit with a cannonball, but I'm perfectly fine now."

*(continued)*

"That's good," says the bartender, "but what about that hook? What the heck happened to your hand?"

"We were in another battle. I boarded a ship and got into a big sword fight. My hand was cut off so I got fitted with a hook. I'm fine, really."

"Well, what about that eye patch?"

"Oh, one day we were at sea and a flock of birds flew over. I looked up and one of them birds pooped in my eye."

"You're kidding," says the bartender. "You couldn't lose an eye just from some bird poop."

"It was my first day with the hook."

## Carpal Tunnel Syndrome

Carpal tunnel syndrome is characterized by pain, numbness, and tingling that occur in one or both hands. It often wakes people from their sleep, leaving them feeling like they have to "shake their hands out" to make the pain and symptoms go away.

This syndrome is caused by the compression of a nerve (the median nerve) as it goes through a narrow tunnel in the wrist formed by the carpal bone, hence the name carpal tunnel syndrome. About a third of people with fibromyalgia have it. All too often the syndrome is treated by surgery. Although this can be effective, it is also expensive and can leave people with residual problems due to the formation of scar tissue that can occur after surgery.

Fortunately, in most cases carpal tunnel syndrome can be relieved without surgery by simply taking vitamin $B_6$ (200 milligrams daily—preferably in a form called pyridoxal-5-phosphate or PYP), thyroid hormone (see information in chapter 5 on thyroid), and wearing a nighttime wrist splint for six weeks. When your hand gets into funny positions while you are sleeping, it stretches and strains the nerve as it goes through your wrist. This is why you wake up in the night with numbness or tingling in your hands. The type of wrist splint to use is called a cock-up wrist splint. It keeps your hand in the neutral position (i.e., the position your hand is in while holding a glass of water), which takes the stress off the nerve. Be sure to wear the splint for at least six weeks while you're sleeping. During those six weeks, also wear it during the day when you can.

# A Few Other Natural Therapies

Here are a few of my favorites.

## BODYWORK

There are many forms of bodywork that can eliminate pain by stretching your tightened muscles. Some excellent ones include Trager, Rolfing, myofascial release, chiropractic treatments, and acupuncture. Some physical therapists are simply too rough, or are unfamiliar with fibromyalgia, and can aggravate symptoms. If any bodywork therapist hurts you, let them know so they can ease back and work more gently. Remember, "No pain, no gain" is a good recipe for hurting yourself. However, a skilled practitioner can effectively help you treat your illness. As you research which techniques and practitioners are right for you, keep these guidelines in mind:

1. Rolfing should be done only by a certified Rolfer with a lot of experience, as some people with minimal training claim that they do Rolfing and can work too aggressively.

2. When talking with a physical therapist, ask if he or she knows how to do Dr. Janet Travell's spray-and-stretch technique. This approach uses a cold spray to briefly block pain, allowing the muscle to be easily and comfortably stretched. I find the best physical therapists for fibromyalgia are those who are familiar with Dr. Travell's work. For those treating pain, I strongly recommend her two-part book series *The Trigger Point Manual*. If you have pelvic pain (vulvodynia or proctalgia), which is common in CFS and fibromyalgia, there is a small subset of physical therapists who specialize in doing muscle release techniques for pelvic pain, and they can be wonderfully helpful. (See "Pelvic Pain Syndromes in Fibromyalgia" below.)

3. Prolotherapy is a technique that may relieve joint pain in people with loose ligaments who can hyperextend their joints and have "loose," elastic skin. The technique consists of injecting weak ligaments with a substance that causes inflammation. The end result of this therapy is to strengthen the ligament, thereby reducing pain.

A very large amount of the pain caused by fibromyalgia comes from tight muscles. The center of the muscle where it bunches up into a tender marble is called a trigger point. Although SHINE gives the muscles the energy they need to release, structural problems can cause persistent localized muscle pain. These can often be helped by simple things that you can do at home to release these muscles. For more information on this, I recommend the book *The Art of Body*

*Maintenance: Winner's Guide to Pain Relief* written by one of my favorite pain specialists, Hal Blatman, M.D.

# Prescription Medications

My preference is to use natural therapies, but I will prescribe prescription medications when needed. In fibromyalgia pain, they can be very helpful. All of the natural therapies I've discussed can be combined with the prescriptions below and can decrease the amount of medication needed while increasing their safety and effectiveness and decreasing side effects.

I do *not* recommend using the Motrin family of medications (NSAIDs) for FMS, as they are minimally effective and dangerous. Fortunately, there are safe and far more effective natural and prescription alternatives. Long-term use of acetaminophen or piracetam, found in Tylenol and many other over-the-counter medications, should be avoided because it depletes your body's glutathione—an amino acid compound that is a critical antioxidant for people with CFS/FMS.

## PRESCRIPTION PAIN CREAMS AND LOTIONS
These can be especially helpful, with virtually no side effects, for small localized areas of severe pain, such as tendinitis or localized neuropathy. I recommend a topical pain cream, which your physician can call into a compounding pharmacy such as Cape Apothecary (410-757-3522) (See Appendix E—"Resources"). These topicals typically include a mix of many pain medications. By rubbing a thin layer

of the lotion or gel into the skin over painful areas two to three times a day for two weeks and then as needed, you can often eliminate your worst pain spots—with virtually no side effects. You can use these products on up to three or four silver-dollar-size areas at a time. Although usually not covered by prescription insurance, they are moderately priced and a 60-gram tube can last a long time.

## PRESCRIPTION ORAL MEDICATIONS

Although there are dozens of medications and other treatments that can be helpful for fibromyalgia pain, here are the ones that I find most effective:

1. *Tramadol (Ultram).* This medication affects both serotonin and endorphin (narcotic) receptors, and is considered minimally addicting, although I've never seen addiction with it in my practice. The recommended regimen is one to two 50-milligram tablets up to three times a day as needed for pain. The most common side effects are nausea and vomiting (when people use more than six tablets a day) and sedation. These effects generally wear off with continued use and can often be avoided altogether by starting with a low dose and slowly working up to the level that most effectively treats your pain.

2. *Gabapentin (Neurontin).* This medication helps nerve pain, central sensitization, pelvic pain, and overall fibromyalgia pain while also helping both sleep and restless leg syndrome. It is also generic and low-cost. So you can see why I hold it in such high regard for fibromyalgia. It is not addictive, although, like any medication, if

high doses are used for long periods, it should be tapered off over time instead of being stopped suddenly. The main side effect is sedation, so I start with a low bedtime dose and then increase as tolerated. Dosing can range anywhere from just 100 milligrams at bedtime to over 3,000 milligrams a day.

3. *Metaxalone (Skelaxin)*. This muscle relaxant has the benefit of not being sedating and generally being very low in side effects in most people. In half of the people it does nothing and in the other half it can help decrease muscle pain. A two-week trial is adequate to see if it will work. The dose is 800 milligrams, one half to one tablet one to four times a day.

4. *Cyclobenzaprine (Flexeril)*. This is a cousin to the medication Elavil that seems to keep most of its benefits and very little of the side effects. It acts as a muscle relaxant and can also be helpful for sleep. The trick is to keep the dose low enough to get the muscle relaxant benefits without the sedating side effects. Interestingly, although the standard dose used to be 10 milligrams three times a day, simply taking 2½ to 5 milligrams at bedtime, and even up to 5 milligrams three times a day, can often be very helpful with minimal side effects.

All four of the above medications can be taken together, and I may give two or three at the first visit for patients to try individually, and then in combination if needed. Because all of these medications are available in low-cost generics (i.e., they are off patent), they cannot be put through the expensive FDA approval process to get an additional recommendation for fibromyalgia.

## AN IMPORTANT NOTE ABOUT PAIN MEDICATIONS

Many people find that they are not able to tolerate any pain medications because of the side effects. When this occurs, it is usually because too high a dose was used initially. Some people tolerate the higher doses without difficulty, so it is not unreasonable to start at the high dose to see if one can get quick pain relief. But if you get side effects that are uncomfortable, instead of abandoning the medication, simply drop to a very low dose, and then slowly work the dose up to the recommended dose as is comfortable.

This works because, unlike narcotic medications, which work best in the beginning and then may lose effect, it takes a while for your body to adapt to the side effects of the medications we are discussing, but the pain-relieving effects tend to increase over time.

In addition, as with many other medications we discuss in this book, most of the benefits occur at lower doses and most of the toxicities occur at higher doses. So it often works best to use a low dose of several medications instead of a very high dose of one. Sometimes, even a very tiny dose can be very helpful for pain.

# Three FDA-Approved
# Medications for Fibromyalgia

These are:

1. *Lyrica (pregabalin).* This is my favorite of the three. It has the benefit of improving sleep, but at doses over 450 milligrams it can increase weight gain and ankle swelling. Although when taken by itself it takes these higher doses to see the optimal effect, when combined with the other treatments we discuss, many people find that simply taking 250 to 300 milligrams at bedtime can help pain and sleep without the side effects.

2. *Cymbalta (duloxetine).* This antidepressant medication raises both serotonin and norepinephrine. It can be especially helpful for nerve pain, tends to be energizing instead of sedating, but can cause *severe* withdrawal symptoms when stopped. I find that if 60 milligrams a day is not helping, increasing the dose is unlikely to add anything besides side effects. This is one of the few medications where it is dangerous to break the pill. So if you want to try a lower dose, have your doctor prescribe a lower-dose tablet.

3. *Savella (milnacipran).* I consider this an expensive form of the medication amitriptyline (Elavil), and have not been especially impressed with its usefulness.

## PELVIC PAIN SYNDROMES
## IN FIBROMYALGIA

These are very common and include:

1. *Interstitial cystitis (IC).* This is a bladder problem characterized by *severe* urinary urgency, frequency, burning, and
   pain. I am not talking about the mild urinary urgency seen
   in fibromyalgia, but rather when it is so severe that people
   want their bladder surgically removed! Once bacterial infections have been ruled out, I add Elavil 10 to 25 milligrams at bedtime plus Neurontin 300 to 900 milligrams at
   bedtime and perhaps during the day as well. I then also
   treat the patient for presumptive candida with oral Diflucan
   for three months. Many supplements including B vitamins
   and vitamin C may aggravate the bladder symptoms in a
   subset of people with IC.
2. *Vulvodynia.* is defined as chronic vulvar itching, burning, and/or pain that is significantly uncomfortable. In this
   condition, vulvar/vaginal pain can either occur only during
   intercourse or be constantly present. In my experience, vulvodynia seems to occur as three main types: neuropathic,
   inflammatory, and muscle pain. I also add bedtime Elavil
   and Neurontin for vulvodynia.
3. *Prostate pain.* Prostate pain is fairly common in men. When
   no infection is found, it is called prostadynia. I suspect that
   prostadynia often occurs because of subtle infections and
   usually improves when these are treated. The bioflavonoid

quercetin 500 milligrams twice a day also decreases prostate symptoms in both prostadynia and prostatitis. I treat with Diflucan for candida first, followed by an extended trial of Cipro or doxycycline if needed.

4. *Endometriosis.* Endometriosis is characterized by abdominal and pelvic pain that is usually worse around the menstrual cycle. It is often associated with other symptoms suggestive of chronic fatigue syndrome and fibromyalgia, such as fatigue, achiness, cognitive dysfunction, and insomnia. For more information, read the book *Endometriosis* by Mary Lou Ballweg and the Endometriosis Association.

I discussed pelvic pain in more detail in my book *Pain Free 1-2-3.*

## Some Other Very Helpful Tips

The natural and pharmacologic treatment options we've discussed will give excellent pain relief in most people. In some cases, however, more aggressive treatment is needed. For more detailed information on pain relief, I recommend my book *Pain Free 1-2-3.*

In addition, here are a couple of simple, yet little-known, treatments that can be very helpful in eliminating even severe chronic pain.

## LOW-DOSE NALTREXONE FOR FIBROMYALGIA PAIN

Good news from the 2012 annual meeting of the American Academy of Pain: a study from researchers at Stanford University School of Medicine showed that a low dose of the drug naltrexone significantly reduced pain in patients with fibromyalgia. The study confirms earlier, similar findings from the same researchers, published in *Pain Medicine* in 2009.

*High* doses (50 to 200 milligrams) of naltrexone can block the effect of heroin and other narcotics—a heroin addict on naltrexone doesn't get high when he takes the drug, which of course helps overcome drug addiction. An injection of naltrexone can also be used to counter a heroin overdose. The sedating action of heroin is blocked, and the addict wakes up. And naltrexone in doses of 50 milligrams is used to help alcoholics stop excessive drinking.

But in *low* doses (3 to 5 milligrams), naltrexone has a very different action—it affects the immune system. In that role, it's been used to treat autoimmune diseases like multiple sclerosis and chronic diseases with an immune component, like cancer and CFS/FMS.

The new study, which was rated among the top six of the many studies presented at the meeting, involved twenty-seven women with fibromyalgia. They took a daily bedtime dose of 4.5 milligrams of naltrexone for twelve weeks and then a placebo for four weeks. Compared to placebo, naltrexone decreased pain by 48.5 percent.

The lead researcher of the study theorizes that the drug

works by suppressing the function of microglia, immune cells in the brain and spinal cord that have been "hypersensitized" and release inflammatory factors that cause pain and other symptoms seen in fibromyalgia.

I've been treating selected CFS/FMS patients with naltrexone for many years. Generally, I give 3.5 to 4.5 milligrams at bedtime. I order it by prescription from a compounding pharmacy (Cape Apothecary (410-757-3522). Your physician can call it in, and if needed the pharmacy can guide your physician in how to prescribe the medicine. An important point is that you need to take it for at least three months for it to work.

It is recommended the person be weaned off all narcotics before beginning the low-dose naltrexone. For more information, see the excellent Web site www.lowdosenaltrexone.org.

## Allodynia—When Even Soft Touch Hurts

Allodynia may occur in more severe cases of fibromyalgia pain. In these cases, even a light touch across the skin may hurt. Although medications for nerve pain may help, in a small subset even these do not. In these cases, I use a medication called Namenda, which inhibits special pain sensors called NMDA pain receptors. The antiviral amantadine (Symmetrel) also blocks NMDA receptors.

In addition, if the pain persists for over three months on the SHINE protocol, it is worth considering a trial of intravenous or subcutaneous infusions of gamma globulin (see page 141). Giving the infusions at a dose of ¼ gram of gamma globulin per pound of body weight three days in a row and then repeating every three to four weeks is one reasonable regimen. Other studies recommend 1 gram gamma globulin per pound over two to five days, and then ½ gram per pound every three weeks. I suspect the higher doses are more effective. Either way, it is very expensive, so make sure it is insurance-covered. Allow the infusions six months to work.

## Wear Wool During Winter

When it's cold outside, wear woolen long underwear. A cold breeze can throw muscles into spasm. So can sweating during a walk if you're overdressed. Woolen long johns will absorb any sweat and wick it away from your skin. Meanwhile, don't forget a scarf and hat. Find wool sheets and pillowcases for your bed as well, as people with fibromyalgia often have night sweats. The wet bedding then causes the muscles to chill and tighten. A beautiful study showed that simply using wool long underwear, sheets, and pillowcases resulted in more pain relief from fibromyalgia than most medications—without any side effects!

### THANK GOD FOR SHEEP! THE BENEFITS OF WOOL

In a 2009 study published in the *JACM* (*Journal of Alternative and Complementary Medicine*), after six weeks, those wearing and sleeping in wool "reported significant improvement in their condition, including a reduction in pain levels, in tender points

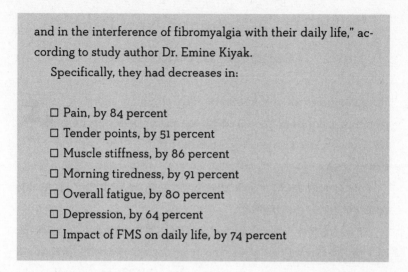

and in the interference of fibromyalgia with their daily life," according to study author Dr. Emine Kiyak.

Specifically, they had decreases in:

☐ Pain, by 84 percent
☐ Tender points, by 51 percent
☐ Muscle stiffness, by 86 percent
☐ Morning tiredness, by 91 percent
☐ Overall fatigue, by 80 percent
☐ Depression, by 64 percent
☐ Impact of FMS on daily life, by 74 percent

Dr. Kiyak called this level of relief "remarkable." I have to agree.

**Narcotics Cause Testosterone Deficiency.** Chronic use of narcotic pain medications like Vicodin, codeine, and oxycodone will routinely cause testosterone deficiency in both men and women. Low testosterone will then cause increased pain. This cycle contributes to the need for ever-increasing doses of narcotics in some people. Because of this, any pain patient who needs chronic narcotic pain medications should have their testosterone levels kept at an optimal level—using only bioidentical testosterone. This not only decreases pain but also improves healing and overall well-being. See chapter 5 for more information.

# HCG—A Dramatic New Pain Treatment Breakthrough

If you've heard of the hormone HCG (human chorionic gonadotropin)—a hormone produced by the placenta during pregnancy—it's probably because you've either heard of, or been on, the HCG diet.

Fortunately, HCG can markedly decrease most kinds of chronic pain—without the dieting.

At the twenty-seventh annual meeting of the American Academy of Pain Medicine, one of the top pain doctors in the United States presented some very positive news about HCG. In a small study, HCG injections provided remarkably effective pain relief for patients with fibromyalgia and others who suffered from severe, intractable pain—so severe that they needed the equivalent of 120 milligrams of morphine a day for pain.

The doctor conducting the study was Forrest Tennant, M.D., from the Veract Intractable Pain Clinic in West Covina, California. Dr. Tennant specializes in treating pain patients whom no one else has been able to help. In this case, he was treating people even he had not been able to help much.

"These were not run-of-the-mill patients," he said. "These were 'the severest of the severe,' what we would term as very intractable patients."

The results? Seven of the eight patients given HCG cut their use of narcotics by 30 percent to 50 percent. Five of the patients said they experienced some pain-free hours. All the patients reported more energy, better concentration, and less depression. And after the year was up, all of them said they wanted to stay on HCG, which was hardly surprising, given the benefits.

Dr. Tennant has put another thirty to forty intractable pain patients on HCG and says, "We're getting positive results in 85 percent to 90 percent of them." He now recommends HCG for all people with chronic severe pain, such as occurs in fibromyalgia.

And I agree with him. I am often starting fibromyalgia patients with chronic severe pain on HCG at their initial visit. An added benefit? Many people are finding marked improvement in their overall CFS/FMS symptoms. In fact, for those who found their CFS improved during pregnancy, or began right after their baby's delivery, HCG may especially improve their overall CFS and fibromyalgia.

HCG is readily available from most compounding pharmacies. This has been a wonderful new development for the treatment of severe chronic pain. Give it three to six months to see the full effect.

## • • •    DOSING HCG FOR PAIN    • • •

As of May 2012, this is Dr. Tennant's recommendation. He adds the HCG to the person's other pain treatments and gives a starting dose of 125 units under the tongue each day or 500 units by subcutaneous injection twice a week. He progressively increases the dose until the patient's pain, energy, sleep, and function improve. The highest dose he has needed was 750 units under the tongue each day. If used by SQ injection, I give 500-1000 units 2-3 times a week. Use the lowest dose that gives the optimal effect. Keep the HCG refrigerated.

. . .

**Soak Your Pain Away.** Add two cups of Epsom salts (which are magnesium salts) to a tub of hot water and then take a delicious soak. The magnesium soaks into your muscles, causing them to relax and even increases magnesium blood levels. This can reduce pain while also helping you to get deep sleep. One caution: for those of you with a low-blood-pressure issue (see page 82—NMH and POTS—orthostatic intolerance), the magnesium can make the blood vessels relax, causing your blood pressure to drop. So be careful the first few times getting out of the tub and have someone give you a hand just to make sure that dizziness is not a problem. Before drying, some people like to do a quick rinse with warm water.

## NEED REHAB?

It is not uncommon for those with chronic pain (emotional or physical) to need help withdrawing from and staying off addictive substances. Unfortunately, most rehab centers don't realize that simply getting the person off the alcohol or drugs—without getting rid of the underlying pains that drove the addiction—is not only unhelpful but usually simply not effective. Meanwhile, many rehab centers try to disempower the person as well as heap a mountain of shame on him or her.

### Noxious and abusive

For a better (and luxury) approach that treats select clients from all around the world, I recommend the Exclusive Hawaii rehab center on the Big Island where I live. Its approach is like a remarkable breath of fresh air, and I am happy to recommend it. See TheExclusiveHawaii.com or call 888.859.2093.

## Important Points

- Most pain can be eliminated.
- Getting eight hours of solid sleep a night, and treating low thyroid function, nutritional deficiencies, and underlying infections (especially yeast), often eliminate the root causes of the pain.
- Try natural and prescription treatments individually and/or in combination, as needed. Dozens of effective ones are available. For more detailed information, see my book *Pain Free 1-2-3* or the longer version, *From Fatigued to Fantastic!* I also recommend the book *The Art of Body Maintenance: Winner's Guide to Pain Relief* (available from www.blatmanpainclinic.com) to learn about structural treatments you can do on your own for pain relief.
- Begin with the herbal mixes Curamin and End Pain one to two tablets of each three times a day for six weeks, then as needed.
- Ultram, Skelaxin, Neurontin, low-dose Flexeril, Lyrica, and Cymbalta are excellent pain medications for CFS/FMS. Avoid Tylenol and Advil family medications.
- Yoga, tai chi, chiropractic, and a host of other treatments can help keep muscles stretched.
- Consider wool sheets, pillowcases, and long underwear and a bedtime hot bath with Epsom salts.

- For those with severe chronic pain, the hormone HCG can be very beneficial.
- Appendix C, "Your SHINE Treatment Worksheet," has a list of the more healthful natural and prescription pain treatments, along with directions for how to use them.

# 10.

# Other Areas to Explore for CFS/FMS

A lthough the SHINE protocol is enough to help most people feel a lot better, sometimes it is not enough and other problems also need to be addressed. Many of these are addressed in more detail in the longer version of *From Fatigued to Fantastic!*, and this is an excellent next step if you are not adequately better with the basics discussed in this "made easy" book. This chapter discusses some of the newer treatment options, while also briefly going through other very helpful areas to explore. I have put "Rx" by those that need a prescription, so you can tell which ones you can do on your own.

## Remember the Basics

When giving lectures, I'm sometimes approached by people who say they've tried *everything* for their CFS or fibromyalgia, but nothing helps. In most cases, I ask them if they've even tried all the basic treatments in the SHINE protocol, such as ribose, the vitamin powder, Ambien, Cortef, Diflucan, or even thyroid treatments. Their answer is usually no.

Occasionally, though, the person is still ill, even after having done SHINE. In this chapter, we'll discuss treatments that can be very helpful in stubborn CFS/FM cases.

If you haven't already done so, do the free "Energy Analysis Program" on the home page at www.endfatigue.com. This will create a SHINE treatment protocol customized to your case, based on your symptoms, and, if available, the pertinent lab tests. Then, if needed, here's what to do next.

# Do Sleep Medications Initially Work for a Few Days or Weeks, and Then Stop Working?

If so, rotate them. For example, if each medication works for only two weeks, then take it (or a mix of a few treatments) for ten days and then go on to the next medication. When you are on the last medication that works, go back to the first one(s). You'll usually find that it is effective again! Another advantage of using *herbal* sleep aids is that it's uncommon to develop a tolerance to them.

## GETTING KIDS AND YOUNG ADULTS WELL—INFORMATION FOR PEOPLE WITH CFS/FMS BETWEEN AGES TEN AND SIXTEEN

If you're under age sixteen, you very likely have postural orthostatic tachycardia syndrome (POTS) or neurally mediated hypotension (NMH)—sort of like low blood pressure—and possibly an allergy to milk proteins. Some doctors do a type of test called the tilt-table test to diagnose NMH and POTS, but I often treat without doing the test first. It's not a bad idea to have it done, but it is expensive and sometimes uncomfortable.

To treat NMH/POTS, your doctor can prescribe the medications fluoxetine (Prozac), midodrine (ProAmatine), fludrocortisone (Florinef, which is modestly effective), and/or methylphenidate (Ritalin) or dextroamphetamine (Dexedrine). Of all of these, Dexedrine and Ritalin are most helpful for those under twenty years of age, but the risk of addiction rises with doses over 20 to 30 milligrams daily. NMH and POTS are discussed in more detail in chapter 5. In addition, the following things can be helpful:

- Avoid sugar. Stevia is a healthy sweetener you can use instead.
- Take the Energy Revitalization System vitamin powder or a similar multivitamin supplement if over ten years old (one-half scoop a day between ages ten and sixteen).

*(continued)*

- Dramatically increase your intake of salt and water. Aim for 8 to 15 grams of salt and one gallon of water each day.
- If you have stomach or bowel symptoms, cut out all milk products and any foods containing casein or caseinate (milk protein) for two to three weeks to see if this helps.
- Consider treatment for candida (see chapter 6).
- If you run frequent fevers (temperatures over 98.8°F), you likely have a hidden infection. A three-to-six-month trial of antibiotics or antivirals, including gamma globulin infusions, should be considered (see chapter 6).
- Consider thyroid treatment with liothyronine (Cytomel).

Fortunately, these simple suggestions help most kids get better.

## More Sleep Treatments

*5-Hydroxy-L-Tryptophan (5-HTP) (natural)*—300 milligrams at night. Naturally stimulates serotonin. Don't take over 200 milligrams a day if you are on serotonin-raising drugs such as antidepressants, tramadol (Ultram), trazodone (Desyrel), milnacipran (Savella), or duloxetine (Cymbalta), and I recommend its use be guided by a holistic health practitioner. 5-HTP can help with sleep, pain, and weight loss. Give it at least three months to work.

*Kava kava* 30 percent extract—250-milligram capsules–one to three capsules at night. Do not use if you have liver inflammation.

*Unisom for Sleep (Doxylamine) or Benadryl*—25 milligrams at night (antihistamines). May also help pain.

*Dimenhydrinate (Dramamine) for motion sickness*—50 milligrams at bedtime.

Rx stands for prescription versus over-the-counter drugs:

*Rx, tizanidine (Zanaflex)*—4 milligrams, one half to two tablets at bedtime for sleep. Stop if it causes nightmares.

*Rx, eszopiclone (Lunesta)*—2 to 3 milligrams at bedtime.

*Rx, doxepin (Sinequen)*—5 to 10 milligrams, one to three capsules at bedtime or doxepin liquid 10 mg/cc. If a lower dose is needed, you can start with one to three drops at night. A powerful antihistamine. Some people get the greatest benefit with the least next-day sedation with a dose of less than 5 milligrams a night.

*Rx, amitriptyline (Elavil)*—10 milligrams, one half to five tablets at bedtime. May cause weight gain or dry mouth. Good for nerve pain and vulvodynia.

*Rx, mirtazapine (Remeron)*—15 milligrams, one to three tablets at bedtime (especially helpful if you feel like you're "hibernating" during the day). Very sedating.

*Rx, tiagabine (Gabitril)*—2 to 6 milligrams at bedtime.

*Rx, pregabalin (Lyrica)*—50 to 300 milligrams at bedtime.

*Rx, quetiapine fumarate (Seroquel XR)*—25 milligrams, one at bedtime (an antischizophrenic medication).

*Rx, olanzapine (Zyprexa)*—10 milligrams, one half to two tablets at bedtime. After six weeks, also helps pain. Causes weight gain (an antischizophrenic medication).

*Rx, GHB (Xyrem)*—an excellent sleep medication in fibromyalgia. Because the DEA claimed that it was being used as a date rape drug, it has gone from being inexpensive and over-the-counter to being tightly regulated and costing approximately $500 a month. If all else fails, this often works very well. Be sure to rinse your mouth well and swallow after taking liquid. If the medication is left to sit on your teeth, it can dissolve your enamel and damage your teeth. I give 6 to 9 cc (4.5 grams) at bedtime and repeat approximately four hours later when you wake up, if needed. The first night you use Xyrem, take it by itself without other sleep meds. The pharmaceutical company will educate you and the doctor on the medication's use. If not for the legal nuisances now attached to it, it would be a first-line sleep treatment, and it is more effective at restoring the deep sleep needed in CFS/FMS than any other natural or prescription sleep aid.

# Hormonal Support

## Rx—CONSIDER A TRIAL OF HIGH-DOSE $T_3$ THYROID HORMONE

If it hasn't been tried, consider a trial of high-dose $T_3$ thyroid hormone. Many people with fibromyalgia have what is called "thyroid receptor resistance," where it takes a very high dose of the active $T_3$ thyroid to get a normal response. It's as if their body is "deaf" and has trouble "hearing" the hormone—and they need very high levels to achieve normal function.

This concept was developed by the late Dr. John Lowe and is discussed in detail in the textbook version of *From Fatigued to Fantastic!* Find somebody specializing in CFS/FMS who is familiar with the use of high-dose $T_3$ to prescribe and monitor this treatment, because high-dose $T_3$ will cause an overactive thyroid if the person is not thyroid receptor resistant!

## STIMULATE HORMONE PRODUCTION WITH PREGNENOLONE

Pregnenolone is a "mother hormone"—the main raw material your body uses to make other hormones, like cortisol, DHEA, estrogen, progesterone, and testosterone. We have found that pregnenolone levels are often low, or low normal, in CFS and fibromyalgia. We suspect that this might be caused by viral infections. Have your level checked—and treat with 10 to 25 milligrams of pregnenolone if you find it's suboptimal.

## Rx—CONSIDER GROWTH HORMONE INJECTIONS

IGF-1 is a biochemical marker for growth hormone (GH)—and we see GH deficiency over and over again in fibromyalgia. If your IGF-1 levels are low or low normal, and the fibromyalgia persists despite SHINE, consider GH injections. These are expensive and require ongoing injections, so this isn't a good early choice for treatment. Good news: exercise, sex, and sleep also raise GH—and I happily recommend all three of these.

## Rx—OXYTOCIN CAN PRODUCE QUICK BENEFITS IN SOME CASES

Oxytocin is an important hypothalamic neurotransmitter, released during orgasm, which is shown to be low in FMS. I suspect a deficiency is present in those who are pale and have cold extremities. The typical dose (administered via intramuscular injection) is 10 units (adding 0.2 cc lidocaine without epinephrine to minimize stinging). If it's going to help, the benefits will begin in forty-five to sixty minutes and will be clear-cut. If the injection works, you can try a sublingual (under the tongue) or nasal spray, made by a compounding pharmacy, to see if there's a similar benefit, but these forms are less effective and more expensive than the injections. The injections can be used daily, or daily as needed.

## IN WOMEN, LOOK FOR PCOS (POLYCYSTIC OVARY SYNDROME)

Ten percent of American women have PCOS, a condition characterized by high blood levels of testosterone and DHEA associated with insulin resistance (blood sugar problems). The symptoms can include acne, increased facial hair, irregular periods, and infertility. If those symptoms are present along with elevated testosterone and DHEA levels, especially if the fasting insulin blood level is over 10, you might have PCOS triggering your CFS/FMS. Treatment consists of:

- The anti-diabetes drug metformin (Rx), at 500 milligrams, one to two times daily. (Metformin can cause vitamin $B_{12}$ deficiency, so be sure to take the Energy Revitalization System vitamin powder with it. Beyond that, it is an excellent and very safe medication.)
- Cortef (Rx), at 10 to 20 milligrams a day, can also improve PCOS.
- Cutting sweets out of your diet—sugar flares PCOS. Add Chromium (GTF or Picolinate 800–1000 mg a day).
- Utilizing one of several birth control pills, which can help regularize the menstrual cycle.

## Treatments for Hidden Infections

### VFEND (Rx, VORICONAZOLE)—ANOTHER PRESCRIPTION ANTIFUNGAL

Have yeast symptoms persisted (e.g., sinusitis, nasal congestion, canker sores—also called aphthous ulcers) despite taking Diflucan? You may have candida resistant to Diflucan, but sensitive to the medication Vfend (very expensive).

### GAMMA GLOBULIN (Rx—IM, IV, OR SQ INJECTION)

Treat with gamma globulin to help clear stubborn infections. If available, use 2 cc by intramuscular injection (IM), once a week for six doses, or 4 cc every other week for three doses. The IM is *much* less expensive than intravenous delivery. Unfortunately, it is often unavailable because it is needed for our soldiers. Otherwise, if covered by your insurance, consider intravenous or subcutaneous gamma globulin. This is basically a solution of antibodies against numerous infections obtained from blood donors. It can be a dramatically effective way to jump-start your immune system, but, again, it is very expensive.

## SYMMETREL (Rx, AMANTADINE)

This old (and cheap!) prescription antiviral can be helpful. But amid the new antivirals that cost $15,000 to $20,000 a year, this pennies-a-day prescription medicine is often forgotten. Ask your doctor about a trial of this medication if you suspect a chronic viral infection. Added benefits? Symmetrel raises dopamine (think more energy) and lowers NMDA (think less pain—especially if allodynia or pain to light touch is present)!

---

### • • •    AN INTRIGUING HYPOTHESIS    • • •

Are CFS and fibromyalgia caused by infections, or by an allergy to the infections?

In an interesting article, Dr. Sarah Myhill, one of my favorite CFS researchers, theorizes that it may not be the viral or bacterial infections themselves causing CFS, but rather our body's own immune reaction to those infections. This is not uncommon in medicine, occurring with rheumatic fever, sarcoidosis, and rheumatoid arthritis.

The role of immune overactivity in illness is highlighted by a recently published study funded by our foundation showing that treating food allergies with NAET (Nambudripad's Allergy Elimination Technique) (see page 129) dramatically improved function in twenty-three of thirty autistic children (versus zero

of thirty improving in the control group). NAET-related techniques also can decrease the reaction to infections, and this
approach has been used by some practitioners to success-
fully treat arthritis. I have personally and repeatedly experienced the symptoms of a cold improving within minutes of
being treated with NAET.

NAET can treat reactions to specific infections. The trick is
knowing what infection(s) to treat for. In addition, NAET does
not routinely include infections in the list of what is treated, so
the practitioner has to specifically consider these and muscle
test for them. Muscle testing is very much an art, and not everyone does it well, so it is good to work with an experienced
practitioner.

An intriguing possibility? It may be possible to treat without
knowing the specific infection involved. This can be done by
muscle testing, and, if the test is weak, treating with NAET
for your:

1. Saliva
2. Blood (a drop collected with the lancets used for diabetes
   blood sugar finger stick testing)
3. Stool
4. Nasal mucus (blow your nose or collect a bit with a Q-tip)

For each of these, a small amount (i.e., a few drops) of the
sample is put in a clean empty glass jar (like a baby food bottle)
and taken with you to the NAET visit. The practitioner tests to
see if it is weak, and also if it is okay to treat (the basic ten al-

*(continued)*

lergen food groups should have been treated first). If so, one of these specimens can be treated at each visit.

Though NAET has been very helpful for treating food and other sensitivities in CFS/FMS, and for treating day-to-day infections, we have not really looked at this for treating the infections in CFS/FMS. We hope to be doing so soon, however. It is possible that instead of using antiviral medications like Valcyte, at a cost of tens of thousands of dollars, or months to years of antibiotics (with the secondary candida), a simple twenty-minute NAET treatment could have the same or better effect!

# Other Nutrients That Can Help Energy

1. NT Factor (pure liposomal glycophospholipids). This was developed by CFS expert Dr. Garth Nicolson. See www.ntfactor.com.
2. Magnesium-potassium aspartate 2,000 milligrams a day.

# Novel Therapies

These are treatments that are not part of the SHINE protocol but can be helpful in some cases.

## CHECK FOR FOOD ALLERGIES

Food allergies can severely aggravate CFS/FMS. To see if food allergies are playing a role, go on a multiple food elimination diet. Detailed information on how to do this can be found at www.vitality 101.com. A wonderful technique to treat food allergies is a specially modified form of acupressure, called NAET. For more information, and a list of the thousands of practitioners worldwide, visit www.naet .com. In addition, many food allergies settle down after you provide adrenal support and treat candida. NAET can be especially helpful for people who are sensitive to most everything.

## CONSIDER MEDICATION-INDUCED FATIGUE

Many medications can cause fatigue as a side effect. If you are on a medication and your fatigue began after you started taking it, talk to your physician about alternative measures or about just stopping it. This is especially important if you are on cholesterol-lowering medications (which can markedly worsen fibromyalgia—and are rarely beneficial unless one has underlying known heart disease) or beta blocker high blood pressure medications (e.g., Inderal [propranolol], Tenormin [atenolol]).

## DETOXIFICATION

Many toxic substances, such as mercury from dental fillings (leave the ones you have alone—just use non-mercury fillings if needed in the future), monosodium glutamate (MSG), aspartame, pesticides, and others too numerous to list, can contribute to CFS/FMS and keep you from healing properly. Many practitioners, especially naturopaths, are well trained in how to use detoxification techniques to rid your body of these toxins. For many people, detoxification may be as simple as sitting in a sauna for thirty to sixty minutes a day. Be sure to drink plenty of water while in the sauna and rinse off immediately afterward so that your skin does not reabsorb the toxins. The dry heat also helps tight muscles to relax and can decrease pain. If you decide to invest in a home sauna, especially if you are chemically sensitive, a far infrared sauna made by Sunlighten (www.sunlighten .com) or High Tech Health (see www.hightechhealth.com) is an excellent choice.

## THE METHYLATION PROTOCOL

The methylation protocol is so promising for people who have persistent symptoms despite SHINE that I have asked two of my favorite people and CFS/FMS researchers to write an article on this. Neil Nathan, M.D., has a practice in northern California. Dr. Rich Van Konynenburg recently died; he was a CFS/FMS advocate with a heart of gold.

Methylation is a biochemical reaction necessary for the building and repair of every cell. The protocol can be very helpful in a subset of CFS patients who don't improve with standard treatment. For more information on the protocol and the supplements that help, see Dr. Neil Nathan's articles at the prohealth.com Web site and read Dr. Nathan's book *On Hope and Healing: For Those Who Have Fallen Through the Medical Cracks*.

While doing the methylation protocol, I would leave off the Energy Revitalization System vitamin powder.

## THE SIMPLIFIED
## METHYLATION PROTOCOL

The simplified methylation protocol is based on the glutathione depletion—methylation cycle block hypothesis for the pathogenesis and pathophysiology of CFS/FMS.

As always, we recommend that anyone on this type of treatment be under the care of a licensed physician. Even though this protocol consists only of nutritional supplements, a small number of people have reported experiencing uncomfortable adverse effects while on it. If this occurs, the protocol should be discontinued.

These are the treatments and how to use them:

1. Neurological Health Formula from Holistic Health, Inc.: This gives overall nutritional support. Begin with one-quarter tablet a day and increase to two tablets daily. Go up to six tablets daily if tolerated.
2. Activated B-12 Guard (Perque): This is a 2,000-microgram lozenge of hydroxocobalamin. Take one lozenge per day, letting it dissolve under your tongue.
3. FolaPro (Metagenics; 800-microgram tablet of L-5-methyltetrahydrofolate): Take one-quarter tablet daily, which amounts to 200 micrograms per day.
4. Folinic acid (800 micrograms of 5-formyltetrahydrofolate): Take one-quarter tablet or one-quarter of the contents of a capsule daily, which amounts to 200 micrograms per day.

*(continued)*

5. Phosphatidyl Serine Complex: Take one softgel capsule daily (can obtain from www.sourcenaturals.com).

All these supplements except #5 can be obtained from www .holisticheal.com. We do not have a financial interest in any of these supplements.

A pill splitter (available from drugstores) will be needed to split tablets.

These supplements can be taken with or without food. Different times of the day work better for different people in regard to effects on sleep. It is best to start with lower dosages than those suggested above and to work up slowly, to make sure they are well tolerated. Some people have found that they are very sensitive to these supplements and can take only much smaller dosages or take them every other day at first. Others find that they need somewhat larger dosages than those suggested.

For those who wish to start the supplements one at a time, we suggest starting with the Neurological Health Formula, then adding the Phosphatidyl Serine Complex, then the $B_{12}$, and finally the folates, with FolaPro last.

Some people have experienced excitotoxicity symptoms when starting this protocol (anxiety, insomnia, and/or a "wired" feeling). Elimination of foods high in glutamate can help. Supplements that may help include GABA, theanine, and magnesium.

Some people have reported experiencing potassium deficiency symptoms while on this protocol. These can include muscle cramps, constipation, arrhythmia, and/or lethargy. If these are experienced, potassium intake should be increased, either with fruits (e.g., bananas or coconut water) and vegetables (e.g., avocados or tomato or V-8 juice), or with potassium supplements.

Most people who have CFS/FMS require additional treatments beyond the simplified methylation protocol. Some of these treatments are discussed in the book *On Hope and Healing: For Those Who Have Fallen Through the Medical Cracks*, by Neil Nathan, M.D., available from Amazon.

A detailed discussion of the glutathione depletion–methylation cycle block hypothesis can be found in the video at http://iaomt.media.fnf.nu/2/skovde_2011_me_kroniskt_trotthetssyndrom/$%7Bweburl%7D.

# HELPFUL ADDITIONAL LAB TESTS

## CHECK FOR CELIAC DISEASE, A GENETIC WHEAT ALLERGY, WITH TWO SIMPLE BLOOD TESTS: ANTI-TRANSGLUTAMINASE IGA AND IGG ANTIBODY

These can be done at most standard labs and give a simple "yes or no" answer. If your test is positive, you'll probably improve dramatically by avoiding gluten, a protein found in wheat. (Important: You must *not* be on a wheat-free diet before the test.)

## CHECK FOR SERUM AMMONIA LEVEL

If it's elevated, which is common, ask your doctor to treat for bacterial bowel infections. Elevated ammonia from bowel infections may also aggravate brain fog. Treatments to improve liver detoxification may also help. We are currently exploring the best approach to take when ammonia levels are elevated and will keep you updated on this in our free e-mail newsletter (from www.endfatigue.com).

## A LONG SHOT

Rituxan (Rx, rituximab)—Balances immune function. Basically, I am adding this because it will likely get a fair bit of attention in the next few years, but I think that the risk and cost relative to the benefits of other options will make this a poor choice.

# Two Simpler Treatments

**Constipated?** Because of bowel infections (especially candida) and low thyroid, some people with CFS/FMS are severely constipated—sometimes only having a bowel movement every five to seven days. This is a quick way to guarantee getting toxic. Begin with simple measures to get at least one bowel movement daily, including optimizing thyroid, eliminating candida overgrowth, eating prunes, taking 500 milligrams magnesium a day and 500 milligrams of vitamin C a day, and then considering other measures as needed. Pantethine supplements of 500 milligrams twice a day as well as chewing *sugar-free* gum can also help stimulate bowel function.

**Don't forget dark chocolate!** Interestingly, research has actually shown that chocolate helps chronic fatigue. Remember, though, it is not a low-calorie food, so keep it to an ounce or less a day. Better yet, sugar-free chocolates can give you the benefits without the sugar blues. Russell Stover makes a good brand that can be found in most supermarkets. Want a treat to die for? Check out the sugar-free section of Abdullah's Candies online!

## The Future Is Hopeful

Although the SHINE protocol can help more than 85 percent of those with CFS/FMS, we are constantly looking for other issues that need to be addressed and treatments that can help. We look forward to achieving our goal of finding effective treatment for everyone!

# 11.

# Am I Crazy? Understanding the Mind-Body Connection

After dealing with an insane medical system, people with CFS/FMS, and even those with simple day-to-day fatigue, often come away wondering if they are crazy.

The simple answer?

NO!

At least not any more than anybody else!

Nonetheless, with all that you have been through, let's take a look at this issue in a little more depth. We have a bad habit in medicine. If a doctor cannot figure out what is wrong with the patient, the doctor brands that patient a "turkey." Imagine calling an electrician because your lights do not work. The electrician checks all the wiring, can't find the problem, and says, "You're crazy. There's nothing wrong with your lights." You flip the switches and they still do not work, but the electrician just says, "I've looked. There's no problem here," and walks out the door. This is analogous to what many CFS/FMS and day-to-day-fatigue patients experience. I apologize on behalf of the medical profession if we've called you crazy just because we cannot determine the cause of your problem. It is inappropriate, abusive, and downright cruel.

Unfortunately, some patients become so frustrated by being told that their CFS/FMS or day-to-day-fatigue is "all in their head" that they are in a catch-22. They feel that if they acknowledge that they also have emotional issues, just like everyone else, they are validating the wacko doctors who say that their illness is all emotional. Rest assured, however, that extensive research proves that CFS/FMS and day-to-day fatigue are real and physical.

One of many studies that proved the CFS and fibromyalgia are real was our placebo-controlled study. This is so because people who received the active SHINE treatment improved dramatically and those receiving placebo did not. If it was "all in your head," the placebo group would have improved as much as the active group. This means that anyone who says it's all in your head is no longer simply a nitwit. Now they are unscientific nitwits. Give yourself permission to be human. You are no more and no less crazy than anyone else.

People often ask if they should get counseling. The simple answer is that, as in any other severe illness, the time to get counseling is if and when you feel like it.

### • • •  HOW TO TELL IF YOU ARE DEPRESSED  • • •

Research has shown that there is a very good way to tell if people are depressed. It is as effective as or more effective than many of the complicated depression questionnaires such as the Beck Depression Inventory.

What is this new high-tech technique?

*(continued)*

Simply ask the person if they are depressed!

Not sure if you're depressed? Here is one more important tip. Ask yourself if you have many interests. If the answer is that you have many interests but are frustrated that you have no energy to do them, then you're probably not depressed. If you have no interests or have lost interest in the interests you used to have, then you likely are depressed and it is good to treat that along with the SHINE protocol. Depression can accompany any severe illness such as cancer, but we wouldn't dream of telling people with cancer that they were simply crazy.

Whether or not you are depressed, you may consider some type of therapist for emotional support and guidance. Be careful whom you choose, however. Make sure "psychotherapist" is one word—not two! Talk to your friends and relatives to find somebody who is good. Your physician may also be an excellent resource.

## The Mind-Body Connection

I suspect that all illnesses have a psychological component. Although highly stressed executives may have a bacterial infection such as *Helicobacter pylori* or excess acid causing their ulcer, it helps to remove the three telephones from their ear while treating the infection and excess acid.

I find that most people with CFS/FMS are mega-type-A overachievers. To some degree, this psychodynamic often applies to day-to-day fatigue as well. We are approval seekers who avoid conflict to avoid losing approval. We often grew up seeking approval from somebody who simply was not going to give it—no matter what. And we take care of everybody except one person—ourselves! Does this remind you at all of yourself?

Being empathic, we also often found ourselves being emotional toxic waste dumps for other people. It almost seems like we would attract every "energy vampire" in town. How do you tell an energy vampire? After an interaction with them, they tell you how much better they feel—and you feel like you were energetically sucked dry!

## The Antidote

So how do you break the psychodynamic? It's pretty straightforward. In fact, it can be summarized in two letters.

N-O.

Learning to use this wonderful word can free you.

Here's how.

When somebody asks you to do something that will take you more than two hours, tell them that you are sorry but the doctor (that's me) told you that I would wring your neck if you took on anything more. Tell him that the answer is probably no, but you'll get back to them in the next twenty-four hours if you change your mind and are able to. Then walk away.

Most often, when you get home you will feel great, like you have dodged a bullet. Since it was left as the answer being no unless you got back to them, you are now off the hook. If, on the other hand, you feel that you really wish you had said yes, and that it would feel really good to do it, you can always call them and change your mind.

Simple—yet effective.

In general, I encourage you to decide to say yes or no based on how things *feel*, more than based on your thoughts. Although it is good to do your homework and check into things, once you have finished this, see how things feel. If it feels good to say yes, then do so. Otherwise say no.

Why is this so? Our mind is a product of our programming as a child. It basically feeds back to us what we were told that we *should* do to be accepted by and get approval from parents, our religious organizations, television, and God knows how many other authority figures. Our feelings, on the other hand, reflect our intuition and also let us know what is authentic to us.

So simply remember the wonderful word "no." It is a wonderfully versatile word. It is a complete sentence. It can be said gracefully or as a very firm "NO!"

There is even a great T-shirt that says, "What part of 'No' didn't you understand?"

## Three Steps to Happiness

Having worked with thousands of severely ill patients over the last thirty-five years, I have found that there are three steps that will leave you feeling happy, no matter how ill you are:

1. *Be authentic with your feelings.* This means to feel all of your feelings, without the need to understand or justify them. When they no longer feel good, let go of them.
2. *Make life a "no-fault" system.* This means No Blame, No

Fault, No Guilt, No Judgment, No Comparing, and No Expectations, on yourself or anyone else. This means you'll be changing habits of thinking. For example, if you find yourself judging somebody, simply drop the judgment in midthought when you notice it. And no judging yourself for judging others.

3. *Learn to keep your attention on what feels good.* We sometimes are given the misconception that keeping attention on problems is more realistic. That is nonsense. Life is like a massive buffet with thousands of options. You can choose to keep your attention on those things that feel good. You'll notice that if a problem truly requires your attention at any given time, it will feel good to focus on it. Otherwise, you're living your life as if you have two hundred TV channels to choose from, but you're only watching the ones you hate—to be "realistic."

For more on this, I invite you to read my e-book *Three Steps to Happiness!: Healing Through Joy.* It will give you the tools that you need to feel great emotionally!

## THE PROBLEM WITH COGNITIVE BEHAVIORAL THERAPY (CBT)

Cognitive behavioral therapy teaches people coping skills and can be very helpful for many crippling illnesses, including cancer, multiple sclerosis, and a host of other conditions. The prob-

*(continued)*

lem occurs when practitioners think that they have to convince the person that the person's illness is not real as part of the CBT. Those practitioners have lost touch with reality and can be quite abusive—even if well-meaning.

Picture the reaction if a CBT practitioner was not only trying to convince people with metastatic cancer that they did not have a real illness but aggressively worked to get legislation passed making it illegal for these people with cancer to get the treatments or insurance coverage they needed and had paid for! This would be considered obscenely abusive, and it is equally inappropriate in CFS and fibromyalgia. On the other hand, many excellent CBT therapists treat their CFS and fibromyalgia patients with respect, helping them to cope by giving them the powerful tools that CBT has to offer—without trying to invalidate their illness.

## Important Points

- CFS, fibromyalgia, and day-to-day fatigue are physical processes with physical causes. However, like most illnesses, they also have psychological components that must be treated.
- If something does not feel good, that is all the justification you need to say "No!"

# 12.

# Losing Weight

Weight gain is a problem for many people, but especially so in those with CFS/FMS. In addition to the myriad other problems you have to bear, two studies of ours found that fibromyalgia and CFS patients have an average weight gain of thirty-two pounds. Because of the metabolic problems that occur in these syndromes, it is almost impossible to lose the extra weight and keep it off until you receive proper treatment. Many of the same metabolic problems are going on in people with day-to-day fatigue as well.

## So What Caused the Weight Gain?

Let's begin with poor sleep. The expression "getting your beauty sleep" actually has a basis in fact. Deep sleep is a major trigger for growth hormone production. Growth hormone stimulates production of muscle (which burns fat) and improves insulin sensitivity (which decreases the tendency to make fat), while also decreasing fibromyalgia symptoms. Thus, getting the eight to nine hours of sleep a night that the human body is meant to have can powerfully contribute to your staying young-looking and trim. Poor sleep also causes lower levels of the hormone leptin, which regulates hunger. Studies have shown that poor sleep is associated with an average six-and-a-half-pound weight gain.

Hormonal problems also play a major role. The thyroid is like your body's gas pedal—regulating how many calories you burn—and low thyroid can dramatically trigger weight gain. The adrenal glands are the body's stress handlers. In the beginning of your illness, chronic stress and depression result in elevated cortisol levels, which can directly cause weight gain. Continuing excessive stress may result in exhaustion of the adrenal glands over time, causing people to crave sugar and eat more than they normally would. This leads to further weight gain.

Infections can also contribute to weight gain. Clinical experience has shown that fungal overgrowth stirs sugar cravings and leads to weight gain. Although we do not know the mechanism for this, we have repeatedly seen excess weight drop off once this overgrowth is treated and eliminated.

Another major problem is carnitine deficiency, a problem that is present in most CFS/FMS patients. Unfortunately, this deficiency forces your body to turn calories into fat and makes it almost impossible to lose fat. Simply taking supplemental carnitine does not help adequately, however, as it does not transfer into cells optimally in this form. I do recommend that people take 1,000 milligrams of *acetyl-L-carnitine* daily for four months, as cells can absorb this form easily, allowing the body to increase energy production and lose weight.

Last but not least, many people with CFS/FMS have insulin resistance—meaning they need high blood levels of insulin to maintain a normal level of blood sugar. Unfortunately, high insulin levels cause your body to pack on the fat!

# So How Can You Go About Treating These Problems So That You Can Lose Weight and Feel Better?

1. Cut down the sugar and simple carbohydrates in your diet and increase your water intake. If your mouth feels parched and you are not taking a medication that causes dry mouth, then you are thirsty and need to drink more water (even if you already drink like a fish).
2. Sleep; Take the treatment needed to get eight to nine hours of solid sleep a night as discussed in chapter 4.
3. Treat low thyroid or adrenal function, if applicable.
4. Treat yeast/candida overgrowth, if present.
5. Get optimum nutritional support. When you are deficient in vitamins or minerals, your body will crave more food than you need, and your metabolism will be sluggish. As mentioned, take 500 to 1,000 milligrams of acetyl-L-carnitine daily along with the Energy Revitalization System.
6. Treat insulin resistance, if present.
7. Avoid medications like Elavil (amitriptyline) that cause weight gain.

It is not unusual for people to shed thirty to fifty pounds simply by treating these metabolic factors.

## HELP WITH SUGAR ADDICTION

Feel like getting off the sugar seems an impossible task? The good news is that once you understand what is driving your sugar addiction and treat it, it becomes much simpler.

There are four main types of sugar addiction, each involving different forces driving the sugar cravings. By treating the underlying causes that are active in your type(s) of addiction, you will find that not only do your sugar cravings go away, but you also will feel dramatically better overall.

People with CFS/FMS often have all four types of sugar addiction, with one cascading into the other. By treating with the information in this book, you'll be able to treat any or all of the four sugar addiction types below:

**Type 1: Hooked on "Energy Loan Shark" drinks.** *Chronically exhausted and hooked on caffeine and sugar for an energy boost.*

**Type 2: Feed Me Now or I'll Kill You.** *When life's stress has exhausted your adrenal glands.*

**Type 3: The Happy Twinkie Hunter.** *Sugar cravings caused by yeast/candida overgrowth.*

**Type 4: Depressed and Craving Carbs.** *Sugar cravings caused around your period, menopause, or andropause.*

For more information on this, I invite you to also read my book *Beat Sugar Addiction Now!*

# 13.

# Finding a Physician, Lab Tests, and Other Helpful Tools

Peple ask me how they can talk their doctor into giving them the treatments they need. In most cases, the answer is that you can't. Most doctors, appropriately enough, will not do the things that they are not properly trained in. This does not make them bad physicians. If you came to me and said, "Dr. Teitelbaum, I would like you to do a heart bypass operation on me," I would say, "I'm sorry, I am not trained in that, and I can't." If you then gave me a copy of a book called *The Bypass Solution* and a scalpel, well, you still would not want me performing surgery on you. This would not make me a bad physician, and your doctor not treating you for CFS/FMS or fatigue does not make them a bad physician, either. The best thing to do is to go to a physician who specializes in treating these complex problems.

## Holistic Physicians

The American Board of Integrative Holistic Medicine has certified more than 1,800 holistic practitioners, and part of their certification often includes the treatments discussed in this book. In addition, more states are recognizing the simple but important reality that naturopaths trained in four-year programs are as competent as physicians and should have the legal right to treat and prescribe based on their training. To find a naturopathic physician who has graduated from a four-year school, see www.naturopathic.org.

Most physicians who know how to help fatigue and CFS/FMS patients are considered holistic. These doctors usually have advanced training in using natural therapies and also spend a lot of time exploring the scientific literature. They also allow the longer visits needed to treat these problems. Unfortunately, most insurance companies will pay well for procedures and surgery but not for a physician to spend time working with the patient. Basically, they often pay less than the physician's overhead for time spent, if you spend more than ten minutes with the person. They also don't cover natural therapies. Because of this, most physicians who can effectively deal with these illnesses cannot participate with insurance. Fortunately, the biggest expense is for lab testing and medications, which are often insurance-covered. So even though the cost to see the physician won't be covered by your insurance, many of the other costs may be.

# When Looking for a Physician, Consider the Following Questions

1. Do they specialize in treating fatigue, CFS, and FMS and recognize these as real and physical conditions?
2. Will they prescribe the medications needed for you to get eight hours of sleep a night?

3. Do they use bioidentical hormones based on your symptoms, even if the tests are normal?
4. Will they treat for candida with Diflucan for six weeks?
5. Do they give nutritional IVs (e.g., Myers' cocktails)?

If the answer to these five questions is yes, you have a physician who is likely to be able to help you.

## • • •   FINDING A HOLISTIC PHYSICIAN   • • •

Holistic doctors are much more likely to know how to help CFS/FMS patients. To find these, I recommend the three organizations below.

### 1. American Board of Integrative Holistic Medicine (ABIHM)

Certifies physicians as having advanced training in the use of natural therapies.

Their Web site lists more than 1,500 physicians throughout the United States.

www.abihm.org

### 2. American College for Advancement in Medicine (ACAM)

P.O. Box 3427
Laguna Hills, CA 92654
www.acam.org

*(continued)*

### 3. American Academy of Naturopathic Physicians (AANP)

www.naturopathic.org

For a list of naturopathic physicians with four-year advanced training. More and more states are recognizing their right to prescribe medications as well as natural therapies.

# More Good News

I am working hard to train as many physicians as I can. I invite you to use our "Physician Finder" at www.endfatigue.com or www.vitality101.com to find health practitioners around the world who have taken the extra time to familiarize themselves with the SHINE protocol. So, whether you have CFS/FMS, simple fatigue, or are over forty-five years old and want a tune-up, the "Physician Finder" is the best place to begin. This list will also include other professionals, such as nutritionists, naturopaths, chiropractors, psychologists, and disability attorneys, who have a special interest in CFS and fibromyalgia. If you have a health practitioner you find to be excellent at treating these conditions, please also invite them to join the list!

# Would You Like a Consultation with Dr. Teitelbaum?

I consult both in person and by phone, treating people with CFS, fibromyalgia, and severe fatigue worldwide. My new patient visits are two to four hours of my one-on-one time, which allow me to prescribe and manage your care, but I also offer one-hour consultations for those who would simply like to discuss their case and get treatment recommendations that they can talk over with their physician.

In addition, I offer ninety-minute "Executive Tune-ups" by phone for those who would like to optimize their energy and vitality. These visits really can help make 50 be the new 30!

For more information, see www.endfatigue.com, e-mail my office at office@endfatigue.com, or call us at 410-573-5389.

# Getting Insurance Coverage for Labs and Medications

As I've noted, most physicians specializing in CFS/FMS do not work with health insurance companies. Nonetheless, I find that if people have prescription coverage, most of the lab testing and medications will be covered. For those of you without prescription insurance coverage who have low incomes (common in CFS/FMS), many, if not most, of the medications you'll need may be supplied for free by the drug companies. For more information on this important option, go to www.pparx.org.

In addition, the price of the same generic medication will routinely vary by over 400 percent from pharmacy to pharmacy, so it pays to compare prices. This can be done easily by going to www .costco.com, then click on "Pharmacy," and then "Price Checker," so you can see what it should cost. You do not have to be a Costco member to get your medications filled there, and their prices are excellent. Another option is to get the medications by mail from Consumer's Discount Pharmacy at 323-461-3606, which also has very low prices.

There are literally over $1 million worth of tests that you can do for CFS and fibromyalgia. On the other hand, I consider very few of these to be actually helpful and worthwhile. Basically, if a test is not likely to affect treatment, I am not likely to recommend it.

Here are the tests that I find to be important in guiding treatment. It is reasonable to do them all at the first visit, but they can also be done in stages if cost is an issue. For those without health insurance, be aware that you can negotiate a 50 percent discount from most labs if you offer to pay at the time the lab tests are drawn and if they don't have to submit to insurance. This must be negotiated *before* they draw your blood; after the test is done you have very little negotiating power.

Tests 1–14 are good for everyone with fatigue (though the reverse $T_3$ can be left off in day-to-day fatigue), and the other tests are for CFS/FMS.

## RECOMMENDED LAB TESTS

### Most important

1. CBC (blood count).
2. General chemistry (include glucose, AST, ALT, calcium, sodium, potassium, and magnesium)
3. ESR (sedimentation rate). In CFS this is usually low. If over 15, I look for autoimmune diseases and infections.
4. Ferritin. This is the best measure for iron levels. If under 60 ng/ml, I give iron (30 to 60 milligrams a day with 60-milligram vitamin C to increase absorption). If above the normal range, hemochromatosis (a genetic iron excess disease) must be considered and ruled out.
5. Vitamin $B_{12}$ level. If under 540 pg/ml, I give a series of ten to fifteen vitamin $B_{12}$ injections. The higher the lab result, the better, so don't worry if it is above "normal."
6. Fasting morning cortisol. *Must* be drawn before 10 a.m., and before eating or drinking anything besides water that morning. If 16 mcg/dl or less, I am likely to give adrenal support.
7. HgBA1C (glycosylated hemoglobin). If 5.3 or less, I am more likely to give adrenal support. If over 5.8, I consider insulin resistance or diabetes.
8. Free $T_4$. If in the lower third of the normal range, I consider thyroid hormone.
9. TSH. If over 2, I consider thyroid hormone. If under .5, if the free $T_4$ is elevated it suggests an overactive thyroid. If

*(continued)*

the free $T_4$ is in the lower third of normal, it suggests low thyroid based on hypothalamic dysfunction.

10. DHEA-S. If under 120 mcg/dl in women or 300 mcg/dl in men, I consider DHEA supplementation. If over 180 µg/dl in women, I consider PCOS (polycystic ovarian syndrome).

11. Reverse $T_3$. If elevated or high normal, it suggests thyroid receptor resistances.

12. Free and total testosterone. If in the lower third of the normal range, suggests need for testosterone supplementation. If elevated in women, consider PCOS.

13. FSH and LH. If elevated in women, suggests estrogen deficiency or menopause. In men, helps determine the cause of low testosterone.

14. Anti-TPO antibody. Screens for Hashimoto's thyroiditis. If elevated, suggests increased need for thyroid hormone, although it can also be elevated with an overactive thyroid.

## Helpful, but More Expensive Tests That Can Wait on the Results of Other Treatments

Ammonia: Screens for bowel bacterial overgrowth and decreased liver detoxification ability.

Pregnenolone: The source hormone for cortisol, testosterone, and others.

IGF-1: If low normal, consider growth hormone if not responsive to other treatments.

*O and P: Stool test for parasites (see chapter 6, "I—Infections: Destroy Your Body's Hidden Invaders"). Do at specialty lab.

*Stool for *Clostridium difficile* (C. *diff.* or toxin): Can do at any lab. Must be a loose stool (i.e., that takes the shape of the specimen cup).

Total IgE: If elevated, suggests allergies are a problem and consider NAET (see chapter 10).

**Anti-Transglutaminase antibody IgG (and perhaps IgA): Screens for celiac disease wheat allergy.

Lyme screen: Sadly, I do not consider any Lyme tests to be reliable.

CMV IgG antibody: If over 4, I consider the possibility of viral reactivation.

HHV-6 IgG antibody: If over 4 (or 1:640 or higher), I consider the possibility of viral reactivation.

Immunoglobulin, quantitative, IgA, IgG, IgM, serum

Immunoglobulin G, subclasses 1-4, serum: If any subclass is low, I consider gamma globulin injections: Gamma globulin injections may cause a severe reaction if IgA levels are low.

Rheumatoid factor (latex fixation): Suggests rheumatoid arthritis or a bacterial infection.

---

*For both stool tests take two Dulcolax tablets if needed to get a watery stool specimen. The sample for the *C. diff.* must be taken to the lab within two hours or frozen.

**Must be eating wheat in the several weeks before the test.

Fighting your physician or insurance company is not a good use of your precious energy. Remember, CFS, fibromyalgia, and other chronic fatigue states are now treatable illnesses. In the long run, you will do best using your energy to find a physician with expertise in treating severe fatigue and CFS/FMS, who wants to work with you to help you recover.

# Other Helpful Tools

Treating fatigue or CFS/FMS can be complicated and time-consuming. In addition to using the worksheet in this book to develop your personalized treatment plan, you can also use the free educational "Energy Analysis Program" at www.endfatigue.com. It will analyze your symptoms and, if available, your patient lab tests to create:

- A list of probable factors contributing to your fatigue, CFS, or fibromyalgia.
- Natural remedies (again, tailored to your specific case) that can help you begin a major part of treatment on your own.
- A prioritized list of the prescription treatments most likely to help you.

In many ways, this program is similar to what you will have created using this book, but it will also analyze your lab tests to further help you determine exactly what you need to do to get well. If your physician is open-minded, you may be able to encourage him or her to give you the treatments you need based on either the computer program or the protocol you filled out while reading this book.

We have finally reached the point where the care you need is available from well-trained physicians. Won't it be nice to have a doctor who knows more than you do?

# Important Points

* It is best to see a physician who is an expert in treating CFS and fibromyalgia, as these are complex syndromes.
* There is a free computerized "Energy Analysis Program" available at www.endfatigue.com that can analyze your symptoms and blood tests to help you determine which treatments are most likely to help you get well.
* There is a CFS/FMS "Physician Finder" at www.vitality101.com and www.endfatigue.com, where you can find practitioners with a special interest in CFS/FMS and optimizing energy worldwide.

I consult both in person and by phone, treating people with CFS, fibromyalgia, and severe fatigue worldwide. In addition, I offer ninety-minute "Executive Tune-ups" by phone for those who would like to optimize their energy and vitality. These visits really can help make 50 be the new 30!

For more information, call 410-573-5389.

In addition, you can sign up for a free e-mail newsletter at www .vitality101.com or www.endfatigue.com that will keep you up to date on the newest developments in treating CFS, fibromyalgia, and day-to-day pain.

# 14.

# Conclusion

The person who says it cannot be done
should not interrupt the person doing it.
—*Chinese proverb*

Old mind-sets are often difficult to change. It took many years for chronic fatigue syndrome and fibromyalgia to be recognized as real and physical processes, and for physicians to even take fatigue seriously. As time goes on and more physicians become aware of what is causing these conditions, patients will no longer have to accept being labeled crazy because of a few physicians' ignorance.

We are entering the next stage.

Fatigue, chronic fatigue syndrome, and fibromyalgia are now treatable. This simple fact needs to be demonstrated and reported over and over again to become accepted by physicians. Over time, it is hoped that even more physicians will learn how to treat, encourage, and support their fatigue patients. Simply ignore those who continue to keep their heads stuck in the sand.

# For Those with CFS/FMS

Meanwhile, although your CFS/FMS has been devastating, even this dark cloud has a silver lining. It has taught you what you do not have to do and has given you space to explore who you truly are. You have earned the right to be yourself.

# For Everyone with Fatigue

As you start feeling better, slowly add activities to your life that make you feel good. If you do something that makes you feel poorly, stop doing it. Joseph Campbell, a world-renowned teacher of the mythology of and paths for personal growth in many diverse cultures, was asked how people can stay true to themselves. Put succinctly, his advice was: "Follow your bliss." Perhaps a "should" led you to become an accountant, doctor, or lawyer, but your bliss truly lies in being an artist, mother, poet, or dancer. Perhaps the opposite is true. If you do what makes you feel happy and excited, you will get yourself on the right track. Whatever you do, however, do not try to make up for lost time by trying to do too much. The few lingering symptoms of your illness will effectively let you know when you are pushing too hard. Recognize that your illness may have been a valuable teacher.

By teaching you to choose the things that feel good to you deep in your heart and soul, and aiding you in letting go of things that don't, this illness will have powerfully taught you to be authentic to who you truly are. Having done this myself, I turned these illnesses into a blessing in my life. Being authentic has not only turned my energy circuit breaker back on but also left me having a life I love—along with abundant energy.

It can do the same for you, giving your CFS and FMS journey a happy ending.

Whether you have day-to-day fatigue, or CFS/fibromyalgia, it's time to get your life back NOW!

Love and Blessings
Dr. T

# • Appendix A •

## Getting Started, and My Ten Favorite Supplements

The key is to remember that your body is having an energy crisis and that it needs two key things to heal:

1. Optimize energy production with SHINE—treating Sleep, Hormones, Infections, Nutrition, and Exercise as able. This will fill your tank with *energy*.
2. Plug the leak in your tank that has been draining your energy. In addition to treating infections, this includes choosing to keep your attention on things that feel good while simply saying no to things (and people) that don't. My *Three Steps to Happiness* e-book can help guide you on how to do this.

For SHINE, the treatment checklist you created while reading this book will offer you an excellent start (see Appendix C). To expand on this, do the free "Energy Analysis Program" at www.end fatigue.com, adding the results of any of the lab tests listed on pages 253–256 that you may have.

The first week, add in the nutritional treatments and the sleep herbals. The second week, add in the Curamin and End Pain for pain. The third week add the over-the-counter hormonal support and the fourth week the probiotics.

If you have CFS/fibromyalgia, make an appointment with me, a physician on my Web site "physician finder," or a holistic practitioner from one of the organizations listed in chapter 13 to work with.

In addition, I would be happy to treat you as well (www.end fatigue.com).

For those of you with CFS/FMS, if they are willing, your family physician may be willing to write for Ambien 10 milligrams plus either Flexeril 2½ milligrams, trazodone 25 to 50 milligrams, or Neurontin 300 milligrams at bedtime for sleep. In addition, they may be willing to write some of the pain medications discussed in chapter 9, as these may all fall within their training. Beyond that, it will be difficult to get the prescription hormonal support and anti-infection treatments unless you have a very open-minded, holistic, or well-educated physician. But often people can start to see a marked improvement even without these.

You now have the tools you need to reclaim your life. For some of you, the information in this book will be all you need and are looking for. For others, though, this will just be enough to whet your appetite. In that case, I invite you to read the full-length *From Fatigued to Fantastic!* Some of you will want to read the book from cover to cover, whereas others will simply use it as a reference text, to read about specific areas (e.g., thyroid, adrenal, candida, viral, or antibiotic-sensitive infections) in much more detail. Again, no "shoulds"! Simply do what feels best to you!

To continue to stay up-to-date on the cutting edge of CFS and

FMS research, I invite you to sign up for my free e-mail newsletter at www.endfatigue.com.

It's time to get your life back NOW!

## MY FAVORITE TEN NUTRITIONAL SUPPLEMENTS

Over the years, people have often asked me for a list of my top 10 supplements—the ones to take if you don't have the money, time, or inclination to take more than a few and you'd like to be able to choose those that give you the most "bang for the buck." I've also included several supplements that are excellent for other health problems, such as heartburn and osteoporosis. These are all available at health food stores and www.end fatigue.com.

The first six are part of what I routinely take, and the last four are in my medicine cabinet to use when needed. These are all awesome!

### Nutritional Supplements

1. Energy Revitalization System vitamin powder (Enzymatic Therapy). One daily scoop of this supplement replaces over thirty-five tablets of supplements—talk about saving money and time! Use one half to one scoop a day—whatever feels best to you.

2. D-Ribose (Corvalen). Use one scoop (5 grams) of powder three times a day for three to six weeks, then two times a

*(continued)*

day for CFS/FMS and one scoop a day for regular fatigue. Most people see a marked boost in energy within three weeks.

3. Coenzyme $Q_{10}$ (Smart $Q_{10}$ by Enzymatic Therapy). Chew a 200-milligram wafer each morning.

4. Vectomega. For fish-oil essential fatty acid support, one a day.

## Sleep

5. Revitalizing Sleep Formula (Enzymatic Therapy). Two to four capsules thirty to sixty minutes before bedtime.

## Anti-Yeast Treatments

6. Acidophilus Pearls Elite (Enzymatic Therapy). One pearl three times per week (Monday, Wednesday, and Friday). For CFS/FMS, one a day for five months, then three times a week.

## Hormonal Support

7. Adrenal Stress End (Enzymatic Therapy). This mix of adrenal glandulars, licorice, and other key nutrients provides outstanding adrenal support. Take one to two capsules every morning (or one to two in the morning and one at noon). I take this during periods of high stress, such as when I am on the lecture circuit.

## Preventing and Treating Infections

8. Pro Boost. One packet dissolved under the tongue three times a day at the first sign of infection and until it clears.

I keep this in my medicine cabinet and carry it with me when traveling.

## Pain—Two Outstanding Herbal Mixes

9. End Pain (Enzymatic Therapy). Contains willow bark, boswellia, and cherry.
10. Curamin (EuroPharma). This is a new and remarkable natural remedy for pain. It contains curcumin, boswellia, nattokinase, and DLPA.

Take one to two tablets of either, or both together, three times a day. It takes two to six weeks to see the full effect, though benefits are often seen in half an hour. These can be taken along with pain medications, allowing the dose of medication to be lowered, or even stopped, over time. Then the dose of the herbal(s) can also be lowered.

For those with fibromyalgia, it's more effective to start with two capsules three times a day of either or both for six weeks.

## Supplements for Specific Problems

The above supplements are helpful for most people, whether with day-to-day fatigue or CFS/FMS. The items below are helpful only if you have the specific problem listed.

## Osteoporosis or Osteopenia (Loss of Bone Density)

OsteoStrong plus Strontium (both by EuroPharma). This combination of products is outstanding for building bone density. The latter contains the mineral strontium, which studies show is

*(continued)*

170 percent more effective than the drug Fosamax for building strong bones—and a whole lot safer and more affordable. OsteoStrong contains bone builders like vitamin D, calcium, vitamin K, and magnesium. If on the vitamin powder in the morning, you can simply add the strontium at bedtime.

## Heartburn, Indigestion, or Reflux

CompleteGest Digestive Enzymes (Enzymatic Therapy). This product is an excellent addition to a regimen to treat and resolve heartburn. Take two capsules with every meal to help digest your food properly. For more detailed information on getting off health-hurting acid blockers like Prilosec, see "How to Get Off Acid Blockers—Naturally" at www.vitality101.com.

Other good techniques include: Sip warm liquids with meals instead of drinking iced drinks (digestive enzymes work poorly at cold temperatures). Take a minute to relax before eating. Chew your food well. Eliminate or minimize coffee (including decaf), aspirin, and alcohol—all of which can worsen heartburn and indigestion. Try drinking four ounces of a diet cola (refrigerator cold) with larger meals, which is as acidic as the hydrochloric acid your stomach makes, to see if this helps digestion.

There are three other excellent natural products that work well together to heal heartburn and indigestion (all by Euro-Pharma):

- Immediate Heartburn Relief chewable antacids. Use instead of plain chewable calcium antacids, which may increase heart attack risk by over 30 percent!

- Gut Soothe (DGL Licorice). This helps heal your stomach.
- Advanced Heartburn Rescue. It contains limonene, which can knock out infections that cause indigestion.

## Anxiety

Calming Balance (Health Freedom Nutrition). This formula is outstanding for anxiety, and though the effects begin within 30 minutes, the calming influences get deeper and deeper over one to four weeks of use. It contains 500 milligrams of vitamin $B_1$, as well as other B vitamins, passionflower, theanine, magnolia, and magnesium. Take one to three capsules, one to three times a day.

## Dry Eyes and Mouth

Hydra 7 (EuroPharma). This essential oil from sea buckthorn berries lubricates dry membranes.

# • Appendix B •

# A Few Study Abstracts of Our Research on Effective Treatment for Chronic Fatigue and Fibromyalgia

The full text of this and a second study on SHINE can be seen at www.vitality101.com.

*Study #1: Published as lead article,* Journal of Chronic Fatigue Syndrome, *Vol. 8, No. 2, 2001, pp. 3–28*

## Effective Treatment of Chronic Fatigue Syndrome and Fibromyalgia—a Randomized, Double-Blind, Placebo-Controlled, Intent-to-Treat Study

*Jacob E. Teitelbaum, M.D.; Barbara Bird, M.T., CLS; Robert M. Greenfield, M.D.; Alan Weiss, M.D.; Larry Muenz, Ph.D.; Laurie Gould, B.S.*

**ABSTRACT. Background:** Hypothalamic dysfunction has been suggested in fibromyalgia (FMS) and chronic fatigue syndrome (CFS). This dysfunction may result in disordered sleep, subclinical hormonal deficiencies, and immunologic changes. Our previously published open trial showed that patients usually improve by using a protocol that treats all the above processes simultaneously. The current study examines this protocol using a randomized, double-blind design with an intent-to-treat analysis.

**Methods:** Seventy-two FMS patients (thirty-eight active; thirty-four placebo; sixty-nine also met CFS criteria) received all active or all placebo therapies as a unified intervention. Patients were treated, as indicated by symptoms and/or lab testing, for: (1) subclinical thyroidal, gonadal, and/or adrenal insufficiency; (2) disordered sleep; (3) suspected NMH; (4) opportunistic infections; and (5) suspected nutritional deficiencies.

**Results:** At the final visit, sixteen active patients were "much better," fourteen "better," two "same," zero "worse," and one "much worse" versus three, nine, eleven, six, and four, respectively, in the placebo group (p<.0001, Cochran-Mantel-Haenszel trend test). Significant improvement in the FMS Impact Questionnaire (FIQ) scores (decreasing from 54.8 to 33.2 versus 51.4 to 47.7) and Analog scores (improving from 176.1 to 310.3 versus 177.1 to 211.9 [both with p<.0001 by random effects regression]), and tender point index (TPI) (31.7 to 15.5 versus 35.0 to 32.3, p<.0001 by baseline adjusted linear model) were seen. Long-term follow-up (mean 1.9 years) of the active group showed continuing and increasing improvement over time, despite patients being able to wean off most treatments.

**Conclusions:** Significantly greater benefits were seen in the active group than in the placebo group for all primary outcomes. Using an integrated treatment approach, effective treatment is now available for CFS/FMS.

*Study #2: Published in* Open Pain Journal *(5), 2012,*
*pp. 32–37* (http://benthamscience.com/open/topainj/
articles/V005/32TOPAINJ.pdf)

---

## Treatment of Chronic Fatigue Syndrome and Fibromyalgia with D-Ribose—An Open-Label, Multicenter Study

*Jacob Teitelbaum, Janelle Jandrain, and Ryan McGrew*

**OBJECTIVES:** Chronic Fatigue Syndrome and Fibromyalgia (CFS/FMS) are debilitating syndromes affecting about 2–4 percent of the population. Although they are heterogeneous conditions associated with many triggers, they appear to have the common pathology of being associated with impaired energy metabolism.

As D-ribose has been shown to increase cellular energy synthesis, and was shown to significantly improve clinical outcomes in CFS/FMS in an earlier study, we hypothesized that giving D-ribose would improve function in CFS/FMS patients.

*Design, Location, and Subjects*: An open-label, unblinded study in which 53 U.S. clinics enrolled 257 patients who had been given a diagnosis of CFS/FMS by a health practitioner.

*Interventions:* All subjects were given D-ribose (Corvalen), a naturally occurring pentose carbohydrate, 5-g TID for 3 weeks.

*Outcome measures*: All patients were assessed at baseline (1 week before treatment), and after 1, 2, & 3 weeks using a Visual Analog Scale (1–7 points) rating energy, sleep, cognitive function, pain and overall well-being.

*Results*: 203 patients completed the 3-week treatment trial.

D-ribose treatment led to both statistically (p<.0001) and clinically highly important average improvements in all categories:

- 61.3 percent increase in energy
- 37 percent increase in overall well-being
- 29.3 percent improvement in sleep
- 30 percent improvement in mental clarity
- 15.6 percent decrease in pain

Improvement began in the first week of treatment, and continued to increase at the end of the 3 weeks of treatment. The D-ribose was well tolerated.

*Conclusions:* In this multicenter study, D-ribose resulted in markedly improved energy levels, sleep, mental clarity, pain relief, and well-being in patients suffering from fibromyalgia and chronic fatigue syndrome; clinicaltrials.gov NCT01108549.

# • Appendix C •

## Your SHINE Protocol Worksheet

### "Short Form" Treatment Protocol

Many of the products mentioned below can also be ordered from 800-333-5287 or www.endfatigue.com, and are available at your local health food store.

Give a treatment six weeks to see its optimal benefits, though they often occur more quickly (e.g., Ribose/Corvalen increased energy by two weeks in most people and an average of 61 percent at three weeks in our study). Side effects, though, if any, will usually occur within the first few days of starting a treatment. So add in one new treatment each one to three days. If a side effect occurs, stop the last two or three treatments for a few days and see if it goes away. If the side effect is acute and worrisome, call your family doctor (or go to the ER) immediately. Do not use if pregnant (except #1, 4, 5, 14, 20, and 23) or drive if sedated. If you have CFS/FMS, it is normal for a woman's periods to be irregular during the first three to four months of treatment as your body returns to a healthy cycle. On average, give yourself three to six months to start feeling better. You can begin to slowly taper off most treatments when you feel well for six months.

Stop things one at a time (e.g., one pill every one to two weeks) so you can see if you still need it. If needed, however, most of these can be used in the long term, although this is usually not necessary. I recommend the vitamin powder (#1) and something for sleep in the long term to maintain optimal vitality.

Some prescriptions can be obtained at a much lower cost from Consumers Discount Drug Company (323-461-3606). Another good source for generic prescription drugs, and to find out what they should cost, is www.costco.com—click on "Pharmacy" and use their price checker. This is especially important if you do not have insurance coverage for medications.

Do not take any treatments below that you are allergic to or that have caused prohibitive side effects. Prescription items have "Rx" after their names. If a recommended (i.e., checked off) treatment has a double asterisk (**) by the number, it is a "most important" treatment; if it has a single asterisk (*), it is an important treatment; and no asterisk means the treatment is helpful but not critical. If you choose to simplify your program, you can begin taking just the double-asterisked items followed by the single-asterisked items and then no-asterisked items that are checked off.

We have listed natural/over-the-counter alternatives for most prescription therapies that can be substituted for and/or added to the prescription ones. We often recommend products made by Enzymatic Therapy and EuroPharma as these have excellent effectiveness, potency, and purity. *Dr. Teitelbaum does not accept money from any pharmaceutical or natural products companies whose products he recommends. He has directed that all his royalties for products he makes be donated to charity.* Only the items that have been checked off as you read this book, and #1 and 2, which I recommend for everyone who wants more energy, are the ones recommended for you, along with any needed pain treatments.

## Nutritional Treatments

### Laying the Foundation

_____ 1. **Energy Revitalization System—Powder (by Enzymatic Therapy): One half to one scoop a day (as feels best) blended with milk, water, or yogurt. This gives a solid foundation for overall nutritional support and replaces more than thirty-five tablets' worth of supplements. If gas or diarrhea occurs, use a lower dose, or divide the daily dose into smaller doses and take two to three times a day. Take #2 (ribose) with it for optimal support.

_____ 2. **D-ribose (Corvalen): One scoop (5 grams) of powder three times a day for three weeks, then two times a day for CFS/FMS or once a day for routine fatigue. If too energizing, take it with food, add Adrenal Stress End (#21), and lower the dose. Effects are usually seen within two to three weeks. This is a key treatment. Take it with #1 (the vitamin powder).

_____ 3. *Coenzyme Q$_{10}$: 200 milligrams once a day. Especially important if taking cholesterol-lowering prescriptions (which I recommend doctors *not* prescribe in CFS/FMS unless the person has known heart disease). Take it with food. I recommend the 200 milligrams Smart Q$_{10}$ chewable wafer by Enzymatic Therapy, which already contains vitamin E to enhance absorption.

_____ 4. *Vectomega: One a day for fish-oil essential fatty acid support (from EuroPharma). Replaces eight capsules of most fish oils. Dry eyes and mouth, pain, inflammation, or depression suggest a need for this.

\_\_\_\_ 5. *Iron

If the ferritin level is under 60, I give 30 to 60 milligrams of iron a day, making sure that the supplement also has at least 100 milligrams of vitamin C to enhance absorption. For those who cannot tolerate iron because of upset stomach or constipation, Floradix makes a liquid iron supplement that has 11 milligrams of iron per dose (take one to two doses a day), is well absorbed, and does not upset the stomach.

Do not take within six hours of thyroid hormone preparations or Cipro (antibiotic), as this can prevent their absorption. Take on an empty stomach (i.e., take between 2 and 6 p.m. on an empty stomach). It is okay to miss up to three doses a week. Stop in four to six months or when your ferritin blood test is over 60. Iron may turn your stool black.

For those with CFS/FMS, also add:

\_\_\_\_ 6. NAC (N-Acetyl-L-Cysteine): 500 to 650 milligrams a day for two to three months. Makes glutathione. Reasonable for anyone with CFS/FMS.

\_\_\_\_ 7. *Acetyl-L-carnitine: 500 milligrams, one capsule once or twice a day for three months.

For Anxiety—Natural Treatments

\_\_\_\_ 8. *Calming Balance from Health Freedom Nutrition: One to three capsules one to three times a day is outstanding for anxiety (the effect increases with one to four weeks of use).

## **Sleeping Aids

For day-to-day fatigue, #9 and 10 will usually be plenty. For CFS/FMS, you will likely also need to add the medications.

Adjust dose as needed to get eight to nine hours of solid sleep without waking or hangover. If unable to find a combination from the treatments below that does this, see the extensive treatment protocol in chapter 10 for many more options. No going to the bathroom if you wake up during the night unless you still have to go five minutes later. Mixing low doses of several treatments is more likely to help you sleep without a hangover than a high dose of one medication. You can take up to the maximum dose of all checked-off treatments simultaneously. Do not drive if you have next-day sedation (adjust your treatment to avoid this). If you have next-day sedation, try taking the treatments (except the Ambien) a few hours before bedtime. The smell of lavender also helps sleep, so consider a bit of lavender oil spray on your pillow or a drop under your nose. Lavender capsules (called Calm Aid by Nature's Way)—take one at bedtime—can also help.

## Foundations
_____ 9. **Revitalizing Sleep Formula (made by Enzymatic Therapy, Integrative Therapeutics): 200 milligrams valerian, 90 milligrams passionflower, 50 milligrams Suntheanine, 30 milligrams hops, 12 milligrams piscidia, and 28 milligrams wild

lettuce. Take two to four capsules each night. If valerian energizes you (occurs in 5 to 10 percent of people), use the other components for sleep.

_____ 10. *Melatonin: ½ milligram at bedtime. This is as effective as higher doses for sleep. Five milligrams at bedtime may decrease nighttime acid reflux, and added to a sleep pillow wedge (see www.hammacher.com) and one half teaspoon baking soda (e.g., Arm & Hammer) taken in four ounces water at bedtime can markedly ease nighttime acid reflux.

_____ 11. *5-HTP (5-Hydroxy-L-Tryptophan): 200 to 400 milligrams at night. Naturally stimulates serotonin. Don't take more than 200 milligrams a day if you are on serotonin-raising drugs such as antidepressants, unless okayed by your health practitioner. Can also help with pain and weight loss. Takes three months to see full effect.

_____ 12. Sleep Tonight (Enzymatic Therapy): If tired all day and then your mind is wide awake at bedtime, this mix of ashwagandha and phosphatidylserine can help by balancing adrenal stress hormone levels. Effects are seen by one week. Take one to two at night.

_____ 13. If you wake between 2 and 4 a.m., take a one ounce high-protein snack (an egg, some meat, or a handful of nuts) to see if this helps. This works by preventing sharp drops in blood sugar during sleep. Also try an acid blocker at bedtime to see if acid reflux is the cause. If yes, take one-half teaspoon baking soda in four ounces of water at bedtime and use a sleep pillow wedge (see www.hammacher .com).

## Sleep Intensive Care

_____ 14. \*\*Zolpidem (Ambien): 10 milligrams—one half to one tablet at bedtime. May be addictive, though we only have seen this at doses over 10 milligrams/night. If you tend to wake during the night, leave one-third to one half of a 5-milligram tablet at bedside and you can take it as needed, crushed between your front teeth and put under your tongue to help you fall right back asleep. Alternatively, you can take Intermezzo to get the same effect at approximately one hundred times the cost.

_____ 15. \* Rx, trazodone (Desyrel): 50 milligrams—one half to two tablets at bedtime.

_____ 16. \* Rx, gabapentin (Neurontin): 300 milligrams—one to two capsules at bedtime. Also helps pain and restless leg syndrome.

_____ 17. \* Rx, cyclobenzaprine (Flexeril): 5 milligrams—one half to two tablets at bedtime. A muscle relaxant. The 2½-milligram dose gives most of the benefits and usually avoids next-day sedation.

## Hormonal Treatments

## Thyroid Support

### *Thyroid Basics*

_____ 18. Tri-Iodine (EuroPharma): 6.25 milligrams a day (or even just three days a week) for two to four months if you have daytime body temperatures under 98.3°F or breast cysts or tenderness. If acne or severe worsening of indigestion, lower the dose or stop. Benefits will be seen within one month, and most find they can stop it after three months. Others need it for the long term, but should have a health practitioner monitor thyroid function.

_____ 19. *BMR Complex (Integrative Therapeutics): This excellent mix of thyroid glandulars, iodine, tyrosine, and other key nutrients is often very helpful for thyroid support. Take one to two capsules two to three times a day.

### *Thyroid Intensive Care*

Thyroid hormone support can be very helpful in many cases of day-to-day fatigue, even if blood tests are normal. In CFS/FMS, I routinely give a trial of thyroid hormone unless the free $T_4$ hormone level is at the upper end of the normal range. The main risks of thyroid treatment are:

Triggering caffeine-like anxiety or palpitations. If this happens, cut back the dose and increase by one half to one tablet each six to eight weeks (as is comfortable) or slower. If you have severe, persistent racing heart, call your family doctor and/or go to the emergency room.

Triggering heart attack. Like exercise, for those who are already at high risk of having a heart attack or severe "racing heart" (atrial fibrillation), thyroid hormone can trigger a cardiac episode. In the long run, though, as with exercise, thyroid much more often markedly decreases the risk of heart disease. If you have chest pain, go to the emergency room and/or call your family doctor. It will likely be chest muscle pain (not dangerous), but with heart attacks, it is *always* better to be safe than sorry. To put it in perspective, I've never seen this happen despite treating many thousands of patients with standard doses of thyroid hormones.

There are several forms of thyroid hormone, and one kind will often work when another does not. A compounded mix of $T_4$ and $T_3$ hormone may be best if your doctor is familiar with these. Do not take thyroid hormone within six hours of iron or calcium supplements or you won't absorb the hormone. It can take three to twelve months to see the thyroid's full benefit.

_____ 20. **Armour thyroid, or a compounded $T_4/T_3$ combination (Rx) 15 to 90 milligrams/day (one half grain = 30 milligrams) (natural thyroid glandular). Sometimes, pure $T_4$ (Synthroid) 25 to 100 micrograms a day works better if the $T_4/T_3$ mix causes edginess. If adrenal support is checked (#21 or 23), begin the Cortef and/or adrenal support one to seven days before starting the thyroid.

## Adrenal Hormones (Glandulars and Support)

Helps your body deal with stress and maintains blood pressure. Also settles down irritability and those "Feed me *now*, or I'll kill you" moments. In addition to helping energy, can save thousands of dollars in marriage counseling and divorce attorney costs!

*Basics*

_____ 21. **Adrenal Stress End (from Enzymatic Therapy or Integrative Therapeutics): One to two capsules each morning (or one to two in the morning and one at noon). If it upsets your stomach, take less or take with food.

_____ 22. *Increase your salt and water intake—a lot. If your mouth and lips are dry, you're dehydrated—drink more water (or herbal tea or lemonade sweetened with stevia; see #26), not sodas or coffee. Celtic Sea Salt is an excellent form to use (www.celticseasalt.com, 800-867-7258).

*Adrenal Intensive Care*

_____ 23. **Cortef (Rx, hydrocortisone): 5-milligram tablets—one half to two and a half tablet(s) at breakfast, one half to one and a half tablet(s) at lunch, and none to one half tablet at 4 p.m. Use the lowest dose that feels the best. Most people find that one to one and a half tablets in the morning and one half to one tablet at noon is optimal. Take it with food if it causes an acid stomach. Do not take more than 15 milligrams a day unless higher doses are markedly beneficial, in which case it is important that you discuss the risks versus benefits with your physician. If taken too late in the day, Cortef can keep you up at night. After nine to eighteen months, you can try to wean off the Cortef (decrease by half a tablet a day every two to six weeks) if you feel okay (or no worse) without it. Compounded sustained-release hydrocortisone is even better (available from Cape

Apothecary, 410-757-3522) if your energy drops in the afternoon.

## Other Hormones

### Bioidentical Hormone Support for Men and Women Going Through Andropause or Menopause

____ 24. *Biest 0.1 to 0.5 milligrams, plus progesterone 30 milligrams, plus testosterone 0 to 1 milligrams all in 1 gram of cream (Rx): Apply 1 gram of skin cream at bedtime. Available from Cape Apothecary (410-757-3522). Vaginal preparations are usually the most effective form.

____ 25. **Testosterone (Rx): Males 25 to 50 milligrams (plus 5 milligrams of progesterone) one to two times a day (less if acne occurs). Rub the cream into an area of thin skin on the abdomen or inner thigh. The cream is available by prescription from Cape Apothecary (410-757-3522) and can be mailed to you. Or Fortesta (Rx): 20 to 70 milligrams a day applied to the thighs. If you do not have prescription insurance, it is best to get the testosterone from a compounding pharmacy as it is much less expensive, and it is okay if your health insurer wants you to use Testim or Androgel instead of the Fortesta. Consider also checking estrogen and DHT levels when you check your testosterone blood levels. If the DHT goes too high it can cause hair loss, which may be prevented by Proscar (Rx) or saw palmetto, 160 milligrams two times a day (but usually suggests the need to lower testosterone dosing). If estrogen goes too high, this can be blocked by Arimidex (Rx): 1 milligram, taking one third of the tablet three times a week.

## Anti-Yeast Treatments
_____ 26. **Candida Basics

**Avoid sweets—this includes sucrose, glucose, fructose, corn syrup, or any other sweets—until your doctor says that it is okay to include them in your diet again. Also, avoid fruit juices, which are naturally sweet. Having one to two fruits a day (the whole fruit as opposed to the juice) is okay. Want to satisfy your sweet tooth? Stevia is an excellent herbal sweetener. A great-tasting one is made by Body Ecology (800-478-3842). Use all you want.

**Acidophilus Milk Bacteria—Pearls Elite (by Enzymatic Therapy): Take one a day for five months. Then consider one a day every other day (e.g., Monday, Wednesday, and Friday) to help maintain a healthy bowel. Do not take within six hours of taking an antibiotic (e.g., take it midday, if you take the antibiotic morning and night). The Pearls Elite form contains 5 billion health-promoting bacteria per pearl. I use Pearls, as otherwise the probiotics are often killed by your stomach acid—rendering them useless. The Pearls are like little "tanks" that protect your probiotic "troops," getting them safely past the stomach acid. The Optima line by Nature's Way is another excellent option.

_____ 27. **Monolaurin/Lauricidin

Monolaurin has been shown to be active against a number of viruses and bacteria, along with having antifungal activity, making it an excellent way to help maintain health.

## How to Take Lauricidin

Take it with or after meals. The mini pellets can be placed in the mouth and swallowed with water. Do not chew or take with hot liquids, or it will taste oily. It can be potent enough against the infections to trigger a die-off reaction at high dose, so you may want to begin slowly, at 750 milligrams (one-quarter blue scoop) or less one to two times daily for a week before increasing the amount. The level can then be increased to 1.5 grams (one half blue scoop) one to two times a day. One container is enough to tell if it will help. Continue it for a total of three to five months for those with candida and day-to-day fatigue, and for one year for those with CFS/FMS.

_____ 28. **Diflucan (Rx, fluconazole): 200 milligrams a day for six weeks. If yeast-related symptoms flare when you start the treatment (called a yeast die-off reaction or Herxheimer), your holistic physician will guide you on adjusting the dose.

## Immune Stimulants

## "Must-Haves" for Your Medicine Cabinet

_____ 29. **Thymic protein (ProBoost): Dissolve the contents of one packet under your tongue—any that is swallowed is destroyed. Take it three times a day at the first sign of any infection until the infection resolves (usually just a day or two). It often knocks out the infection very quickly. For the chronic infections seen in CFS/FMS, however, it takes three months to see the full effect.

_____ 30. *Zinc lozenges: Suck on 20 milligrams of zinc acetate lozenges four times a day when you have a sore throat or cold to help it go away more quickly and decrease the symptoms.

_____ 31. Discuss antiviral agents such as Valcyte or Isoprinosine with a CFS/FMS specialist, and take #27.

_____ 32. Discuss antibiotic treatment with a CFS/FMS specialist.

## Water Filters

_____ 33. *Water filters: Many water filters, except those that use reverse osmosis, are not optimally effective. I recommend the ones available from my favorite water expert, Bren Jacobson (www.jacobsonhealth.com or 410-224-4877). They decrease the risk of reinfection and remove chemicals and contaminants from your water.

## Chronic and Acute Sinusitis

_____ 34. **Sinusitis nose spray (Rx, by prescription from Cape Apothecary, 410-757-3522). It contains an antifungal, xylitol, Bactroban, and beclamethasone. Use one to two sprays in each nostril twice a day for six to twelve weeks.

## Food and Other Sensitivities

_____ 35. **NAET: Wonderful for elimination of sensitivities/allergies (see www.naet.com for more information).

## Pain Treatments

*The natural treatments can be substituted for or added to the prescription pain medications.* If side effects occur, they can often be avoided by starting with a low dose and raising it every three to seven days as your body gets used to the medication. It may take two to six weeks for a treatment to start working.

## BASICS—Natural Pain Therapies

The natural treatments can be substituted for or added to the prescription pain medications. It may take two to six weeks for a treatment to start working.

### Natural Pain Therapies

_____ 36. *End Pain (by Enzymatic Therapy) or Pain Formula (Integrative Therapeutics):
    Contains willow bark, boswellia, and cherry. Take two tablets three times a day. It takes two to six weeks for maximum effect.

_____ 37. *Curamin (by EuroPharma): This herbal mix is remarkable for pain in general. It contains a special form of curcumin, which has ~700 percent the absorption of others, DLPA, boswellia, and nattokinase. Take one to two capsules three times a day until the pain resolves or six weeks (whichever comes first), and then the dose can be lowered. Amazing!

_____ 38. Take a hot bath with Epsom salts. Add two cups of Epsom salts (magnesium sulfate) to a tub of hot water and feel your muscles relax as the magnesium soaks into them.

_____ 39. For nerve pain, take lipoic acid 300 milligrams two times a
day. An excellent mix for nerve pain is called Healthy Feet
and Nerves (by EuroPharma). It may take three to six
months to see the full effect. Treatments 1, 3, and 7 above
also help nerve pain.

## Pain Intensive Care

These Can Be Added to the Natural Therapies for localized small
areas of especially problematic pain.

### *Topical treatments*

_____ 40. Topical Pain Formula (Rx): Rub a pea-size amount onto
painful areas three times a day as needed (Cape Apothecary, 410-757-3522). You can use this on up to three or
four "silver dollar"–size areas at a time. Good for most
kinds of localized pain, and with virtually no side effects.

## A Special Treatment for Chronic Pain

_____ 41. **HCG hormone (Rx): Begin with an injection of 500 units
SQ twice a week for two weeks, which can be increased to
1,000 units twice a week until you see optimal improvements in pain or two months (whichever comes first). Then
you can try the SL under the tongue drops (or you may
simply begin with the drops instead of the injection). For
the drops, give 125 units SL a day, increasing the dose to
the optimal level (up to 750 units a day). This is highly rec-

ommended for anybody with severe chronic pain requiring ongoing long-term pain medications. HCG must be kept refrigerated. This is available from Cape Apothecary (410-757-3522) by prescription.

## Oral Medications for FMS Pain

Although there are dozens of others (see my book *Pain Free 1-2-3*), these are the ones I find most helpful:

_____ 42. *Ultram (Rx, tramadol): 50 milligrams, one to two tablets up to four times a day as needed for pain. Side effects are less with four or fewer tablets a day. May cause nausea/vomiting. Caution: May very rarely cause seizures or raise serotonin too high when combined with antidepressants.

_____ 43. *Neurontin (Rx, gabapentin): 100 to 900 milligrams two to four times a day (to a maximum of 3,600 milligrams a day). Cut back and increase by 100 milligrams a day each four to five days if it causes any uncomfortable or unusual neurologic symptoms or excessive sedation. Begin with 100 to 300 milligrams at night, slowly increase to 300 to 900 milligrams three times a day as is comfortable. In some, pain relief is immediate; in others, it can take a minimum of 1,200 milligrams a day. You can go up to 3,600 milligrams a day.

**OR**

_____ 44. *Lyrica (pregabalin); 150 milligrams, one or two capsules twice a day. It can be helpful when other treatments don't work. I prefer to keep the total daily dose to no more than 300 mg a day, as most of the side effects are lower at this dosing. It may sometimes take up to 600 mg a day to see optimal effects, though.

## Muscle Relaxants

_____ 45. *Flexeril (Rx, cyclobenzaprine): 3 to 10 milligrams at bedtime and three to four times a day. Muscle relaxant. Low doses (e.g., 5 mg) cause less sedation and are still very effective.

_____ 46. *Skelaxin (Rx, metaxalone): 800 milligrams four times a day as needed for pain. This is usually nonsedating.

# • Appendix D •

## Some Other Helpful Books by Jacob Teitelbaum, M.D.

1. Want more information on CFS, fibromyalgia, or severe fatigue? Looking for more detailed information on an area you've read about here? Read the number one best-selling book of all time on fatigue, CFS, and fibromyalgia.

   *From Fatigued to Fantastic!* (Avery/Penguin, 2007) is the authoritative textbook on these topics, and also includes much more detailed information on specialized areas of the SHINE protocol as well as other treatments. *The Fatigue and Fibromyalgia Solution* was written at the request of thousands of people who said that they wanted a simple and easy-to-understand version. Having read this, *From Fatigued to Fantastic!* is for those of you who are now ready for more detailed and in-depth information. It even includes a chapter written in "medicalese" that you can give your physicians, if they want detailed information on how to treat people with CFS and fibromyalgia.

2. *Three Steps to Happiness!: Healing Through Joy* (Deva Press, 2012). This simple e-book available on Amazon (or at endfatigue.com

for the PDF download) will teach you how to feel happy when you choose to be and get a life you love.

3. *Pain Free 1-2-3* (McGraw-Hill, 2006). For those with chronic pain, this book will teach you how to be pain-free using a mix of natural and prescription therapies tailored to the type of pain you have.

4. *Real Cause, Real Cure* (Rodale Press, 2012). This book is like a natural owner's manual for your body. In easy-to-understand language, it goes through the nine key areas for maintaining and optimizing health, and discusses over one hundred illnesses, telling you what to do if your body "breaks down."

5. *Beat Sugar Addiction Now!* (Fairwinds, 2010). For you sugar addicts reading this, it will show you how to come off of sugar easily, while still satisfying your sweet tooth.

6. *Beat Sugar Addiction Now Cookbook* (Fairwinds, 2012). Offers delicious sugar-free recipes.

7. *Beat Sugar Addiction Now for Kids* (Fairwinds, 2012). Teaches adults how to help their children break the sugar habit.

I also recommend the free iPhone and Android app Cures A–Z.

## • Appendix E •

## Other Resources

**Physicians Specializing in Chronic Fatigue Syndrome and Fibromyalgia**
See the CFS/FMS "Physician Finder" at www.endfatigue.com.

**Make an Appointment with Dr. T!**
I treat fatigue, CFS, and fibromyalgia patients from all over the world in person and by phone consultations, and will be happy to help you recover your health and fight fatigue. In addition, I offer ninety-minute "Executive Tune-ups" by phone for those who would like to optimize their energy and vitality. These visits really can help make 50 be the new 30! For more information, see www.vitality101.com, e-mail office@endfatigue.com, and/or call 410-573-5389.

**Dr. Teitelbaum's Web Sites**
www.endfatigue.com
For our supplement shop and articles on optimizing health. Get an extra 20 percent off our already very low prices by using our "auto ship program."

www.vitality101.com

For thousands of articles on treating hundreds of health problems—
with a special focus on CFS and fibromyalgia.

## Online Energy Analysis Program

The Energy Analysis Program (see www.endfatigue.com) can analyze
your medical history (and key laboratory test results, if available) to
determine the underlying problems contributing to your fatigue or
fibromyalgia, and offer recommendations tailored to your case. This
will allow you to begin the natural parts of the protocol on your own
and will assist and support your doctor in giving you the best possible
care. More good news? It's free! It is also growing to help you optimize your total health!

I also invite you to sign up for free e-mail newsletters.

## Compounding Pharmacies

There are numerous excellent compounding pharmacies worldwide.
One of my favorites is:

*Cape Apothecary*
1384 Cape Saint Claire Rd.
Annapolis, MD 21409
800-248-5978; 410-757-3522; 410-974-1788
www.capedrugs.com

They make a wide array of prescription compounded hormones and
other treatments and do an especially excellent job making inject-
able medications, including vitamin $B_{12}$ and HCG, which are then

mailed to the patient. The pharmacist Thomas J. Wilson, Pharm.D., is excellent and can help answer questions you and your physician may have.

To find a compounding Pharmacy near you, see the International Academy of Compounding Pharmacists (IACP), www.iacprx.org.

## For a Wide Selection of High-Quality Supplements

*Enzymatic Therapy*

800-783-2286

www.enzymatictherapy.com

Produces many excellent products, including the Fatigued to Fantastic! product line, which I developed. This line includes Fatigued to Fantastic! Energy Revitalization System vitamin powder and B complex; Fatigued to Fantastic! Daily Energy B Complex; End Pain; Adrenal Stress End; and Revitalizing Sleep Formula. Enzymatic Therapy products can be found in most health food stores, as well as at www.endfatigue.com.

*EuroPharma*

866-598-5487

www.europharmausa.com

This company was founded by Terry Lemerond, who's been at the head of innovation in the natural products industry for decades. Their products include Curamin, which is likely the most powerful natural pain remedy in history! Using new natural technologies, they have developed ways to dramatically increase the absorption of nutrients, so that you don't have to take handfuls of pills every day. For example, their fish-oil supplement Vectomega supplies the effect of eight large fish-oil capsules in one tablet. They have also revolutionized the herb curcumin, using the highly absorbed BCM 95 in products such as Cura Med, Healthy Knees and Joints, and Bos-Cur. They also make Tri-Iodine, OsteoStrong, Strontium, Hydra 7 (for dry eyes and mouth), Healthy Nerves and Feet, and a suite of three excellent digestion products (Immediate Heartburn Relief, Gut Soothe, and Advanced Heartburn Rescue). To find the cutting-edge of natural health, just look for Terry!

## Support and Self-Help Groups

There are numerous excellent self-help groups in the CFS and fibromyalgia community.

Here are a few of my favorites:

### 1. Fibromyalgia Coalition International

www.fibrocoalition.org

Yvonne Keeney is a tireless patient advocate for those suffering from fibromyalgia, and this organization has a wide range of resources.

### 2. Thyroid Support

www.thyroid-info.com

Mary Shomon is my favorite patient advocate in the whole world for those with thyroid diseases. Her thyroid newsletter ("Sticking Out Our Necks") is simply awesome. She has written numerous books and also offers personalized thyroid coaching.

## Help for Chronic Sinusitis

*Sinus Survival by Robert Ivker, M.D.*
www.fullyalivemedicine.com
His book *Sinus Survival* is a must-read for those with sinus problems. For those living in the Boulder, Colorado, area, I am excited to note that he is now seeing patients again. Dr. Ivker embodies the heart of what it means to be a holistic physician.

# • Index •

# About the Author

Jacob Teitelbaum, M.D., is the author of the popular free iPhone and Android application "Cures A–Z," and of the best-selling book *From Fatigued to Fantastic!*, *Pain Free 1-2-3—A Proven Program for Eliminating Chronic Pain Now*, the Beat Sugar Addiction NOW! series, and *Real Cause, Real Cure*. He is the lead author of four studies of effective treatment for fibromyalgia and chronic fatigue syndrome. Dr. Teitelbaum does frequent media appearances, including Good Morning, America; CNN; Fox News Channel; the Dr. Oz Show; and Oprah and Friends. He lives in Kona, Hawaii. His Web site: www.EndFatigue.com.